Slow down

down

Go

Fasting

Unlocking Health, Clarity, and Transformation through Fasting

SLOW DOWN, GO FASTING

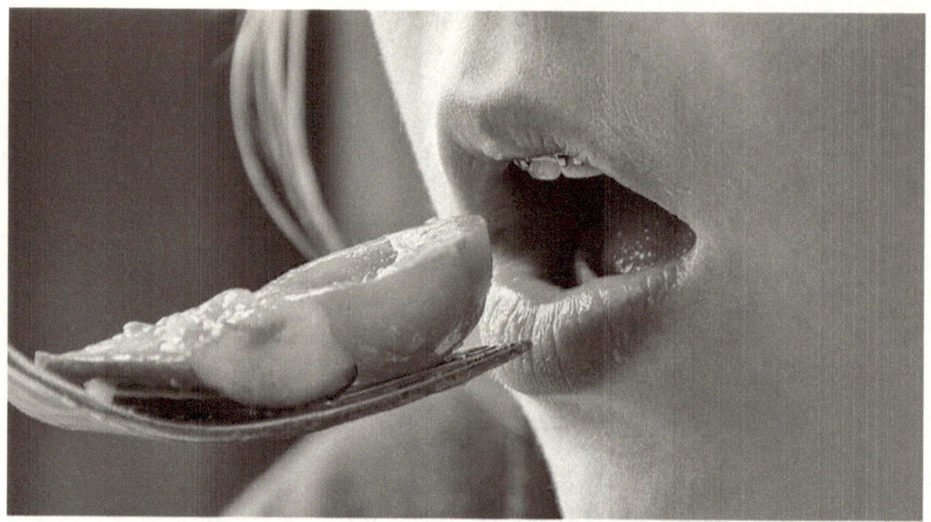

In a world that never stops, discover the art of slowing down to unlock boundless health, clarity, and transformation. "Slow Down, Go Fasting" is your comprehensive guide to embracing the ancient practice of fasting in the modern age. Beyond weight loss, this book takes you on a journey that delves into the science of fasting, the myriad health benefits it offers, and the profound impact it can have on your mental and spiritual well-being.

You'll explore a range of fasting methods and learn how to incorporate fasting into your lifestyle. Through personal stories, expert insights, and practical tips, you'll gain the tools to embark on a transformative path toward balance, vitality, and well-being. This book is an invitation to reclaim your life, align with your true self, and unearth the wisdom of slowing down through the power of fasting. If you seek a life filled with clarity, wellness, and spiritual connection, this book is your compass on this extraordinary journey of taking control of your life.

SLOW DOWN, GO FASTING

SLOW DOWN, GO FASTING

SLOW DOWN, GO FASTING

SLOW DOWN, GO FASTING

Introduction:

He who buries his head deep into a nosebag full of food cannot hope to see the invisible world. -- Al-Ghazali

In a world that constantly races forward, where the demands of daily life keep us perpetually on the move, there's a quiet revolution happening. It's a movement that beckons us to pause, to reflect, and to savor the profound beauty of stillness.

It's time to "Slow Down, and Go Fasting."

This book is your invitation to embark on a transformative journey, one that encourages you to break free from the chaos and embrace the power of fasting. Fasting is not just a practice; it's a philosophy, a way of life, and a path to self-discovery. It's an opportunity to take a step back from the frenzy of modern existence and reconnect with your body, mind, and soul.

The title, "Slow Down, Go Fasting," embodies the essence of this journey. It's a gentle nudge to decelerate, to find solace in simplicity, and to rekindle a profound connection with the rhythms of your own being. Fasting becomes the medium through which you experience this transformation.

In the pages that follow, we'll explore the science behind fasting, delve into a variety of fasting methods, and unearth the incredible health benefits it offers. But this book goes beyond the physical; it delves into the spiritual, the mental, and the emotional aspects of fasting. It's an exploration of the power of intention, mindfulness, and self-discovery.

SLOW DOWN, GO FASTING

Fasting is not about deprivation; it's about liberation. It's about breaking free from the shackles of constant consumption and finding the richness of life in the spaces in between. It's about enhancing your vitality, achieving mental clarity, and connecting with the deepest layers of your consciousness.

With "Slow Down, Go Fasting," you're embarking on a voyage of healing, of rejuvenation, and of awakening. The journey may not always be easy, but it is profound. It is a journey that will empower you to discover your fullest potential and lead a life that's in tune with your innermost self.

So, are you ready to embark on this extraordinary journey of slowing down and going fasting?

Let the adventure begin, and may it lead you to a life filled with balance, vitality, and well-being.

-

-

Chapter 1: Setting the Stage

The Importance of Nutrition and Fasting - Your Journey Begins: What to Expect from your Body and this Book

"Fasting is the greatest remedy—the physician within." — Paracelsus

Fasting: A Journey into Our Ancient Roots and Modern Wellness

Fasting, as a practice, is as old as the human story itself. If we could journey back in time, we'd find our ancient ancestors, the hunters and gatherers, occasionally embracing fasting as a necessity. Picture it: a cold, icy winter, where sustenance was scarce. In those harsh conditions, they relied on sporadic meals like the occasional dead animal or digging for roots in the frozen earth. When food was scarce, they slowed down their metabolism, a biological response shared, to a smaller extent, with hibernating creatures like bears. Fasting, in its essence, is deeply woven into our genetic tapestry. It's a reminder of our ancestors' adaptability and resilience, traits that are still encoded within us, waiting to be awakened.

Fast forward to the new millennium, and fasting has seen a resurgence in popularity. What drives this revival? It's propelled by a growing awareness that fasting may hold the key to unlocking numerous facets of human health. Yet, despite its newfound acclaim, fasting remains somewhat alien to conventional medicine.

SLOW DOWN, GO FASTING

The relationship between fasting and medical science has been historically complex, marked by skepticism and sometimes even discord. This dynamic may seem like a recent development, but it's not entirely new.

Fasting isn't just a clinical concept or a health trend; it's a journey into our own ancient roots and a path toward modern wellness. In this book, we will explore the intricate interplay between this age-old practice and contemporary science, guiding you on a transformative journey that spans millennia. We'll dive deep into the science behind fasting, various fasting methodologies, health benefits, and the art of incorporating fasting into your daily life. Along the way, you'll discover that fasting has the potential to awaken incredible human capabilities that may have lain dormant for too long.

As we embark on this journey together, remember that your experience with fasting will be unique. Fasting isn't just about what you do or don't eat; it's a process that intertwines with your own story, goals, and aspirations. Your personal journey through these pages begins now, and the wisdom you gain here can shape your understanding of health, well-being, and the untapped potential that fasting may hold for you.

Importance of Fasting

Fasting is a practice that has been part of human history for centuries, but in today's world, its significance has been rediscovered. Fasting is not just a trend or a fad diet; it's a lifestyle that can transform your health, both physically and mentally. In this chapter, we will explore the profound importance of fasting, helping you understand why it's worth considering as a part of your wellness journey.

What to Expect?

Before delving into the world of fasting, it's essential to set clear expectations. Fasting is not a one-size-fits-all solution, and your experience will depend on various factors, including your goals, body type, and the specific fasting method you choose. Throughout this book, we will provide you with a wealth of information, practical tips, and insights to help you navigate your fasting journey. You can expect to gain a comprehensive understanding of how fasting works, its potential benefits, and the pitfalls to avoid.

Who Is Fasting For?

Fasting is for anyone seeking to improve their overall health and well-being. It's a versatile practice that can be adapted to various lifestyles and goals. Whether you want to lose weight, boost your mental clarity, enhance your longevity, or address specific health concerns, fasting can be a valuable tool in your arsenal.

Who Should Not Do It?

While fasting can be transformative for many, it's not suitable for everyone. If you have any underlying medical conditions, it's crucial to consult with a healthcare professional before embarking on a fasting journey. Conditions such as diabetes, eating disorders, and certain metabolic disorders may require special considerations.

Additionally, pregnant or breastfeeding individuals should approach fasting with caution, as it can have significant impacts on both the mother and the developing child.

Always prioritize your safety and well-being. If you are taking prescription medications, consult your doctor before fasting, as adjustments may be necessary to avoid potential complications.

If you're new to fasting, consider starting with shorter fasts, such as intermittent fasting, and gradually work your way up to more extended fasting periods. This gradual approach allows your body to adapt and can reduce the risk of adverse effects.

Remember, this book is intended to be informative, but it's not a substitute for professional medical advice. Your health is a priority, so consult with a healthcare expert to determine whether fasting is a suitable choice for you and to receive personalized guidance.

As you explore the world of fasting, keep in mind that knowledge and preparation are your allies. Fasting can be a powerful and life-changing practice, but it's essential to embark on this journey responsibly and with a full understanding of its benefits and potential risks. In the chapters that follow, we will delve deeper into the science of fasting, the various fasting methods, and practical tips to make your fasting experience safe and successful.

Chapter 2: My Journey with Fasting: From Rebellious Runaway to Fasting Enthusiast

"Fasting is the first principle of medicine; fast and see the strength of the spirit reveal itself."

— Rumi

My encounter with fasting has been nothing short of intense. Picture a rebellious 19-year-old runaway in the bustling heart of New Delhi, navigating life as a struggling rock 'n' roll musician. Money was scarce, and days without a proper meal were not uncommon. In those moments, I'd cling to whatever sustenance I could find—perhaps a piece of fruit, a timely visit to a friend's house during lunch, or the dreaded yet reliable trip to a city relative's home where I could feast like royalty for a day before plunging back into the urban jungle. This was life in all its raw uncertainty, including the ebb and flow of food.

My journey followed a cyclical rhythm. There were times when abundance graced my life, and other moments when hunger and quiet contemplation became my companions. Strangely, I found comfort in that companionship; I made friends with hunger. It was during these periods that I realized I wasn't getting sick frequently. Save for a vague memory of bronchitis, which I suspect was due to a misguided attempt to fit in by taking up smoking among friends, my health remained remarkably robust.

As a late bloomer to smoking, starting around 21, I would normally consume a pack of cigarettes a day. However, during fasting phases, my relationship with cigarettes took a peculiar turn. Lighting one up after breakfast, I'd extinguish it after a few puffs, snipping off the charred tip with scissors. Hours later, I'd indulge in a couple more puffs. But by the third day of fasting, the very thought of a cigarette became repulsive. These early experiences with fasting were instinctual; I had yet to comprehend its nuances.

In Indian culture, fasting is a living tradition, deeply woven into everyday life. It finds expression in rituals like "karvachauth," where women abstain from food throughout the day until they can witness the moon's reflection alongside their husband's image in a water-filled dish. Other festivals like Ramadan also feature fasting. Yet, the curious aspect is that while these practices endure, few extol the virtues of fasting, even though our forebears seemed to grasp its benefits intuitively.

Reflecting back, I realize that what sustained me during those days in the city was my ability to transition seamlessly between times of plenty and moments of scarcity. In retrospect, this mirrors the way our hunter-gatherer ancestors must have navigated their worlds.

Today, over three decades later, I still harbor an affinity for fasting. The sensation of hunger, the act of purposeful self-denial, it brings me a sense of comfort. It's a peculiar joy that I cherish, even if my wife, a polar opposite, finds it challenging to skip a single meal.

The journey that began with youthful rebellion has evolved into a lifelong fascination with the art of fasting. This book is an exploration of the knowledge and wisdom I've acquired on this incredible journey, and it's my pleasure to share it with you.

Personal Insights: Beyond the Documented Benefits of Fasting

While the documented benefits of fasting are undoubtedly impressive, my personal journey has revealed additional, subtle rewards that seldom find their way into the scientific literature.

First and foremost, my health has seen remarkable resilience through fasting. I've observed that I rarely fall ill, and when I do, it's a fleeting affair, lasting no more than a day or so. It's as if my body, accustomed to the rhythms of fasting, has learned to protect itself with unwavering vigilance.

In recent years, my fasting repertoire has expanded to encompass a range of approaches. Intermittent fasting, in particular, has become a part of my weekly routine, with several dinners skipped to allow my body a period of rest and rejuvenation. But it's the seasonal fasting rituals that truly stand out.

As the warm embrace of spring ushers in new beginnings and the gentle farewell of autumn invites introspection, I commit to three-day fasts. It's a time when I reflect on the cyclical nature of life and embrace the cleansing power of fasting.

SLOW DOWN, GO FASTING

Yet, the most noteworthy of all is the grand fast that unfurls like a sacred tradition in my life—the post-Christmas fasting. It's a culinary odyssey that commences right after the splendid feast of Christmas lunch and continues through the jubilant celebrations until the dawn of the new year.

During this time, my home became a hub of social activity. My wife's family, cousins, and children gather, and the kitchen becomes a whirlwind of delectable creations, laughter, and the joyful chaos of festivities. To the outsider, it may seem like a challenging ordeal to abstain while being surrounded by the tantalizing aroma of sumptuous delicacies. The truth is, it is indeed a challenge, but it's one I willingly embrace.

It's during these moments, when the table is laden with dishes that evoke nostalgic memories and temptations beckon from all corners, that I've experienced the true test of my willpower. There have been moments when I've brought a morsel to my mouth, only to promptly expel it. I recall a particularly vivid memory from one such episode during a water fast.

My younger son had left a spoonful of luscious blueberry jam on the kitchen counter. It was an irresistible sight. Without a second thought, I let the jam-laden spoon enter my mouth. Time seemed to slow down, and as my tongue touched the jam, a rush of sweetness enveloped my senses. The temptation to savor it fully was overwhelming, and I allowed myself a brief moment of indulgence before resolutely spitting it out into the compost.

In that seemingly insignificant act, I discovered a profound testament to my inner strength and a marker of my commitment. It was a moment of choice, and I chose to honor the fasting journey.

SLOW DOWN, GO FASTING

While the jam was lost, what I gained was a deep understanding of my capacity to overcome even the sweetest of temptations.

These experiences, beyond the realm of documented benefits, are the treasures of fasting—a testament to the strength of will and the journey of self-discovery that each fasting practice unveils.

I would like to share this poem that i wrote, during one of those fasts. which sums up my experience after a profound seven day fast:

Awakened by Stillness

In stillness, I embarked on a quest,
A journey of the soul, a noble test.
Fasting's grace and meditation's balm,
In silence and solitude, I found calm.

As I shed the weight of worldly cares,
A metamorphosis, my spirit wears.
Through empty hours and hunger's grip,
I found a path to my soul's true ship.

The mirror revealed a different me,
Eyes clearer, a heart more free.
Inward changes, profound and deep,
Awakening from a restless sleep.

Fasting cleansed, like a river's flow,
My body, my mind, a radiant glow.
Meditation, a key to self-discovery,
Revealing my purpose, my soul's recovery.

SLOW DOWN, GO FASTING

Through patience and will, I emerged anew,
Transformed by the practices I drew.
Self-improvement, a lifelong quest,
Fasting and meditation, my dearest guests.

In stillness and hunger, I found my might,
In meditation's embrace, I saw the light.
Transformed, I stand, my spirit whole,
A journey of self, my heart and soul.

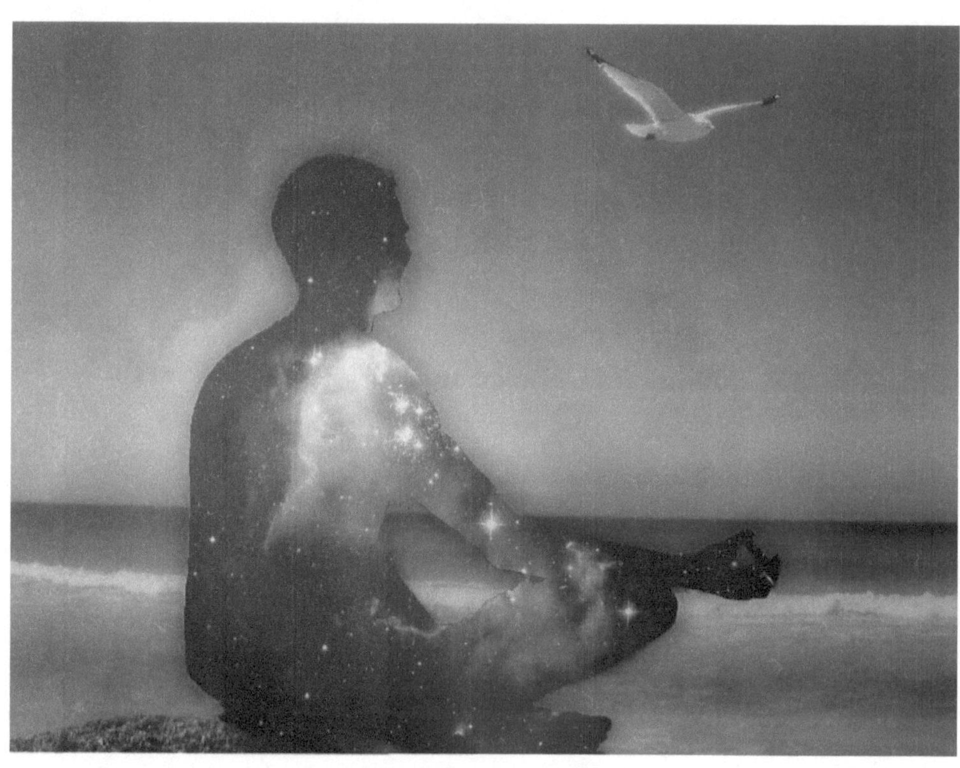

Chapter 3: The Science Behind Fasting

Understanding the Basics: What Happens When You Fast - Fasting vs. Dieting: Key Differences

Fasting is, first and foremost, an exercise for identifying and managing adversity in all its forms. With faith, in full conscience, fasting calls women and men to an extra degree of self-awareness. --Tariq Ramadan

Understanding the Basics: What Happens When You Fast?

Fasting is not just a temporary departure from our regular eating habits; it's a profound physiological shift that takes place within your body. To grasp the essence of fasting, we must dive into the intricate science that governs it. So, let's break it down step by step.

The Physiology of Fasting: A Cellular Symphony

When you embark on a fasting journey, your body enters a state known as "ketosis." During this phase, your primary source of energy shifts from carbohydrates to fat. To understand this, imagine your body as a hybrid car. In your everyday life, you predominantly run on gasoline (carbohydrates). However, when you fast, you switch to an electric mode (fat) for energy. Here's how it unfolds:

1. Glycogen Depletion: Your body's first order of business is to burn through its glycogen stores, a form of stored glucose in the liver and muscles. As these reserves deplete, you transition to the fat-burning mode.

2. Ketone Production: With glycogen levels running low, your liver starts producing ketones, which are molecules generated from the breakdown of fat. Ketones become the primary fuel source for your body during fasting.

3. Fat Breakdown: As you continue fasting, your body begins breaking down adipose tissue (body fat) to release fatty acids, which are then converted into more ketones for energy. This process is what makes fasting an effective approach for weight loss.

4. Autophagy: Fasting also triggers a process called autophagy, where your cells clean the house. They remove damaged or malfunctioning components, promoting cellular renewal and overall health.

Fasting vs. Dieting: Key Differences

Fasting is often compared to traditional diets, but there are significant distinctions that set them apart. While both approaches can lead to weight loss, fasting offers unique advantages. Let's explore these differences:

SLOW DOWN, GO FASTING

1. Insulin Levels: During fasting, insulin levels drop significantly, which enhances your body's ability to burn fat. In contrast, most diets don't have the same impact on insulin.

2. Simplicity: Fasting is straightforward; you eat during specific windows and abstain during others. Diets, on the other hand, can be complex and often involve calorie counting or food restrictions.

3. Metabolic Effects: Fasting can boost your metabolic rate, while long-term dieting can potentially slow it down. This means that, with fasting, you can burn more calories, even at rest.

4. Cellular Benefits: Fasting's effect on autophagy is a significant health advantage. Diets typically don't trigger this cellular cleaning process to the same extent.

Scientific Studies Examples:

The science behind fasting isn't just theoretical; it's backed by a growing body of scientific research. Let's explore a few noteworthy studies that shed light on fasting's benefits:

1. The Nobel Prize-Winning Autophagy Study: In 2016, Yoshinori Ohsumi was awarded the Nobel Prize in Physiology or Medicine for his discoveries related to autophagy, a process that fasting significantly stimulates. His work underscores the fundamental role autophagy plays in cellular health.

2. Intermittent Fasting and Weight Loss: A study published in the journal JAMA Internal Medicine in 2019 compared time-restricted

feeding (a form of intermittent fasting) with traditional calorie restriction. It found that those practicing time-restricted feeding lost more weight and experienced better metabolic outcomes.

3. Fasting and Longevity: Research in animals, such as a study on mice published in the journal Cell Metabolism, has shown that periodic fasting can extend lifespan and improve overall health.

These are just a few examples of the numerous scientific studies that highlight the power of fasting. As we delve deeper into this book, we'll continue to explore the science behind fasting, its various forms, and how it can unlock remarkable health benefits. Whether you're intrigued by weight loss, improved metabolism, or cellular rejuvenation, fasting has the potential to transform your health in ways that diets simply can't replicate.

Chapter 4: Types of Fasting

Intermittent Fasting: A Gentle Start - Water Fasting: The Deep Cleanse - Juice Fasting: A Nutrient-Packed Approach - Extended Fasting: Pushing the Limits - Fasting Mimicking Diets: The New Frontier

"The mind is not a vessel to be filled, but a fire to be kindled." — Plutarch

Fasting is not a one-size-fits-all practice. There are various approaches, each with its unique characteristics and benefits. In this chapter, we'll explore five primary types of fasting and help you determine which one might align best with your goals and lifestyle.

Intermittent Fasting: A Gentle Start

Intermittent fasting (IF) is like dipping your toes into the world of fasting. It's a flexible approach that alternates between periods of eating and fasting. Here are some common methods of intermittent fasting:

- 16/8 Method: This method involves fasting for 16 hours and eating during an 8-hour window. It's a popular choice and can be easily integrated into your daily routine.

- 5:2 Diet: With this approach, you eat regularly for five days a week and restrict calorie intake to around 500-600 calories on the other two non-consecutive days.

- Eat-Stop-Eat: In this method, you fast for a full 24 hours once or twice a week.

Intermittent fasting is an excellent starting point for many because it's not overly restrictive and offers several health benefits, including weight loss, improved insulin sensitivity, and increased autophagy.

Water Fasting: The Deep Cleanse

Water fasting is often seen as the ultimate detox and reset for your body. During a water fast, you consume only water, completely abstaining from food and other beverages. The benefits of water fasting include:

- Autophagy Intensification: Water fasting is a powerful driver of autophagy, leading to cellular rejuvenation.

- Rapid Weight Loss: Due to a significant calorie deficit, you can experience fast and dramatic weight loss.

- Mental Clarity: Many people report enhanced mental clarity and focus during water fasts.

- Detoxification: It's believed to help the body flush out toxins.

Water fasting, however, is not for beginners. It's a rigorous practice that should be done with caution and under medical supervision for extended periods.

Juice Fasting: A Nutrient-Packed Approach

Juice fasting is a more gentle fasting method that involves consuming freshly squeezed fruit and vegetable juices. It provides vital nutrients while giving your digestive system a break. Benefits of juice fasting include:

- Nutrient Boost: You flood your body with vitamins, minerals, and antioxidants.

- Digestive Rest: It's easier on your digestive system than solid food.

- Improved Hydration: You stay well-hydrated, which is crucial for overall health.

Juice fasting can be a great option if you're looking for a balanced way to detox and rejuvenate your body without the intensity of water fasting.

Extended Fasting: Pushing the Limits

Extended fasting refers to fasts that go beyond 48 hours, typically ranging from several days to even weeks. It's an approach that requires a high level of commitment and should be approached with caution. Benefits of extended fasting include:

- Maximum Autophagy: Extended fasting maximizes the cellular cleansing process.

- Significant Weight Loss: It can lead to substantial weight loss and fat reduction.

- Potential Health Improvements: Some studies suggest extended fasts may benefit certain health conditions.

Extended fasting is not recommended for beginners, and medical supervision is crucial, especially for longer fasts.

Fasting Mimicking Diets: The New Frontier

Fasting mimicking diets (FMDs) are a recent innovation that provides some of the benefits of fasting while allowing for small, carefully controlled food intake. These diets typically involve consuming specific foods in specific quantities to mimic fasting effects. Benefits of FMDs include:

- A More Sustainable Approach: FMDs offer fasting benefits with less dietary disruption.

- Enhanced Compliance: They can be easier for some people to adhere to.

- Potential Health Improvements: Early research suggests that FMDs may offer health benefits similar to traditional fasting.

In this chapter, we've scratched the surface of the fasting world, introducing you to five distinct fasting methods. Each has its merits, and as you continue your journey through this book, you'll discover in greater detail how these methods can be integrated into your life and contribute to your health and well-being.

Chapter 5: Mono-Diet Fasting: Embracing the Power of One

Fasting is not nearly as deadly as feasting.-- J. Harold Smith

Fasting is a journey with many paths, and sometimes, the road less traveled leads to unexpected and unique destinations. Mono-diet fasting, an unconventional but increasingly popular approach, centers around the consumption of a single food item, typically a fruit or vegetable, for a defined period. In this chapter, we explore the fascinating world of mono-diet fasting, its benefits, and considerations, as well as practical tips to help you embark on a journey that revolves around the power of one.

Understanding Mono-Diet Fasting:

Mono-diet fasting is rooted in the idea of simplicity and minimalism in nutrition. Instead of a diverse array of foods, you'll nourish your body with just one particular item, whether it's watermelon, bananas, apples, grapes, or even potatoes. The focus here is on the purity and unique properties of the chosen food, along with the potential health benefits it offers.

Benefits of Mono-Diet Fasting:

This specialized fasting method offers several potential benefits:

1. Digestive Ease: Consuming a single food can ease the digestive process as it's relatively straightforward for the body to process and absorb.

2. Nutritional Focus: The chosen food item is often nutritionally dense and can provide essential vitamins, minerals, and other nutrients.

3. Hydration: Many mono-diet fasts involve fruits with high water content, contributing to hydration during the fasting period.

4. Simplicity: Mono-diet fasting can be simpler to plan and execute compared to more complex fasting regimens.

Planning Your Mono-Diet Fast:

Before undertaking a mono-diet fast, it's crucial to consider factors like duration, the choice of food, and any potential health considerations. We'll delve into how to structure your fast, select the right food item, and prepare for a successful experience.

Safety Considerations:

While mono-diet fasting can be a valuable experience, it's important to ensure that you're meeting your nutritional needs and that the chosen food item aligns with your health goals and dietary restrictions. We'll provide guidance on how to do this safely.

A Journey of One: My Personal experience with mono diet

Mono-diet fasting, with its focus on the power of one food, is a testament to the simplicity and purity of fasting. Whether you're curious about mono-diet fasting or seeking a new fasting experience, this chapter serves as your guide to understanding and embarking on a fasting journey that revolves around the incredible power of one.

There are various fasting regimens that involve consuming only one specific fruit or plant, often referred to as "mono-diet" fasting. These specialized fasts are believed to offer unique benefits and can be an interesting approach for those looking to explore fasting beyond traditional methods. Here are a few examples:

1. Watermelon Fast: Watermelon fasting involves primarily consuming watermelon for a designated period. Watermelon is hydrating, low in calories, and rich in vitamins and minerals, making it a popular choice for short-term fasting.

2. Banana Island: Banana fasting, sometimes called "Banana Island," focuses on consuming primarily bananas. Bananas are a good source of potassium and provide natural energy.

3. Lemonade Fast (Master Cleanse): This fast is centered around a homemade lemonade made from fresh lemon juice, pure maple syrup, and cayenne pepper. It's designed to detoxify the body and is often done for a few days.

4. Apple Fast: An apple fast involves consuming primarily apples for a specified period. Apples are a good source of fiber and can promote digestive health.

5. Grapes Fast (Grape Cure): The grape fast, also known as the "Grape Cure," focuses on consuming grapes, particularly dark grapes. Grapes are rich in antioxidants and believed to have detoxifying properties.

6. Potato Diet: Although not strictly a fruit, some people undertake a potato diet, consuming only potatoes for an extended period. Potatoes provide essential nutrients and can be a source of sustainable energy.

7. Juice Fasting: While not limited to a single fruit, juice fasting typically involves drinking freshly squeezed fruit and vegetable juices for a specified time. This approach allows for a variety of flavors and nutrients.

8. Single Vegetable Fast: You can also create fasting regimens centered around a specific vegetable, such as cucumber or celery. These vegetables are hydrating and low in calories.

Mono-diet fasting can offer simplicity and may be more palatable to some individuals due to the limited variety of foods. However, it's essential to plan these fasts carefully and ensure that you're meeting your nutritional needs. Consulting with a healthcare professional or nutritionist before attempting a specialized mono-diet fast is advisable, as it can help you make informed choices and ensure your safety during the fasting period.

Specialized Fasting: The Grapefruit Juice Fast

While many fasting methods have garnered attention for their various health benefits, there exists a unique and lesser-known approach— the Grapefruit Juice Fast. This specialized fasting regimen has gained popularity for its potential to detoxify the body, boost metabolism, and support weight loss.

The Grapefruit Juice Fast involves consuming freshly squeezed grapefruit juice as the primary source of nutrition for a specified period. Often recommended as a short-term cleanse, this fasting method has generated interest due to the unique properties of grapefruit.

Grapefruit is renowned for its high vitamin C content and numerous antioxidants. It's also a rich source of phytochemicals, particularly limonoids and flavonoids, which have been linked to various health benefits. These compounds are believed to aid in detoxification and offer protection against certain chronic diseases.

The Potential Benefits:
  - Detoxification: The high antioxidant content of grapefruit may assist in neutralizing harmful free radicals and promoting the removal of toxins from the body.

  - Weight Management: Some proponents of the Grapefruit Juice Fast suggest that the juice can help curb appetite and support weight loss efforts.

  - Digestive Health: The natural acidity of grapefruit may aid in digestion and help maintain a healthy gut.

- Metabolic Boost: Certain studies have explored the idea that grapefruit can influence metabolism and insulin sensitivity.

- Hydration: As with any fasting regimen, adequate hydration is essential. Grapefruit juice can contribute to your daily fluid intake, helping to maintain proper bodily functions.

The Grapefruit Juice Fast in Practice

Before embarking on a Grapefruit Juice Fast, it's essential to consider a few key points:

- Duration: Typically, this fast is relatively short-term, lasting from a few days to a week. Extended periods of grapefruit juice fasting may require medical supervision.

- Fresh Juice: It's crucial to use freshly squeezed grapefruit juice to maximize its nutritional benefits.

- Balanced Approach: Some practitioners combine grapefruit juice fasting with light, whole foods to ensure a more balanced intake of nutrients.

- Potential Risks: While grapefruit juice offers various health benefits, it can interact with certain medications, so it's advisable to consult a healthcare professional before starting this fast.

In this chapter, we explore the Grapefruit Juice Fast in detail, examining its potential benefits, safety considerations, and practical tips for incorporating it into your fasting routine. We also share personal stories of individuals who have found success and rejuvenation through this specialized fasting method. Whether you're intrigued by the detoxifying properties of grapefruit or seeking a new approach to your fasting journey, the Grapefruit Juice Fast may offer unique insights and rewards.

Chapter 6: Health Benefits of Fasting

Weight Loss and Metabolism - Cellular Autophagy: The Body's Recycling System - Improved Insulin Sensitivity - Mental Clarity and Cognitive Benefits - Fasting and Longevity - Detoxification: Separating Myth from Reality

"Fasting is the greatest remedy, the physician within." — Paracelsus

Fasting isn't just about abstaining from food; it's a transformative practice that can lead to numerous health benefits. In this chapter, we will delve into the remarkable advantages of fasting, from weight loss to mental clarity and even its potential impact on longevity.

Weight Loss and Metabolism

One of the most noticeable and sought-after benefits of fasting is weight loss. When you fast, your body taps into its fat stores for energy, leading to a caloric deficit that promotes fat reduction. Fasting can also boost your metabolic rate, allowing you to burn more calories even at rest. Whether you're looking to shed a few pounds or embark on a more profound transformation, fasting can be a powerful tool in your weight management journey.

Cellular Autophagy: The Body's Recycling System

Autophagy, often referred to as the body's recycling system, is a central player in fasting's health benefits. During fasting, your cells undergo a cleaning process, breaking down and removing damaged or malfunctioning components. This not only enhances cell function but also contributes to overall well-being. Autophagy is believed to play a crucial role in preventing various diseases and promoting longevity.

Improved Insulin Sensitivity

Fasting can have a remarkable impact on your body's sensitivity to insulin, a hormone that regulates blood sugar levels. By reducing insulin resistance, fasting can be a valuable approach for those at risk of or already dealing with type 2 diabetes. It's not just about managing diabetes; improved insulin sensitivity can lead to better energy utilization and overall metabolic health.

Mental Clarity and Cognitive Benefits

Fasting isn't just about physical well-being; it can also sharpen your mental acuity. Many fasters report heightened mental clarity, improved focus, and enhanced cognitive function during fasting. The brain's ability to access ketones as an energy source is thought to play a role in this cognitive boost.

Fasting and Longevity

Fasting's connection to longevity has been a topic of considerable research and debate. Studies in animals have shown that periodic fasting can extend lifespan and improve overall health. While the exact mechanisms are still being explored, it's clear that fasting has the potential to influence the aging process and promote a longer, healthier life.

Detoxification: Separating Myth from Reality

Detoxification is a term often associated with fasting, and while fasting does support the body's natural detoxification processes, it's essential to separate fact from myth. Fasting can aid in the removal of toxins, but it's not a miraculous cleanse that will eliminate all your body's impurities. Instead, fasting supports the liver and other organs in their ongoing detoxification functions.

In this chapter, we've scratched the surface of fasting's multifaceted health benefits. As we delve further into this book, we'll explore each of these benefits in greater detail, providing you with a comprehensive understanding of how fasting can improve your well-being. Whether you're looking to optimize your metabolism, enhance your mental clarity, or potentially extend your years, fasting has the potential to unlock a world of health benefits.

Chapter 7: Getting Started with Fasting

Pre-Fasting Preparation: What You Need to Know - Choosing the Right Fasting Method for You - Setting Realistic Goals - Fasting Safety: What to Watch For

"The spirit is willing, but the flesh is weak." — *The Bible (Matthew 26:41)*

Starting a fasting journey is an exciting and transformative step, but it's crucial to begin with the right knowledge and preparation. In this chapter, we'll guide you through the essential aspects of beginning your fasting experience.

Pre-Fasting Preparation: What You Need to Know

Before you dive into fasting, it's essential to understand what you're getting into. Here's what you need to know:

1. Consult Your Healthcare Provider: If you have any underlying medical conditions or are taking prescription medications, consult with a healthcare professional to ensure fasting is safe and suitable for you.

2. Educate Yourself: Learn about the fasting method you plan to follow. Understand its rules, potential benefits, and any possible side effects.

3. Gather Supplies: Depending on the type of fasting you choose, you may need specific supplies, like fresh fruits and vegetables for juice fasting or essential electrolytes for longer fasts.

4. Set Clear Goals: Determine your reasons for fasting, whether it's weight loss, improved health, or spiritual growth. Your goals will guide your fasting journey.

Choosing the Right Fasting Method for You

Fasting is not one-size-fits-all, and the method you choose should align with your lifestyle and goals. Here's a brief overview of the primary methods:

- Intermittent Fasting: Ideal for beginners, it offers flexibility and various approaches to suit your schedule.

- Water Fasting: A deep cleanse but not recommended for newcomers; it requires careful preparation and medical supervision for extended fasts.

- Juice Fasting: A nutrient-packed approach that provides essential vitamins and minerals; it's suitable for those seeking a balanced detox.

- Extended Fasting: A more challenging but potentially rewarding option for those with experience and medical guidance.

- Fasting Mimicking Diets: A novel approach that mimics fasting effects with carefully planned meals, offering benefits and easier compliance.

Setting Realistic Goals

Your fasting journey should be guided by realistic and achievable goals. Whether you aim to lose a specific amount of weight, improve your health markers, or experience mental clarity, setting clear objectives will help you stay motivated and track your progress.

Consider breaking down your goals into smaller milestones. For instance, if your ultimate goal is to lose 20 pounds, celebrate each 5-pound loss as a significant achievement.

Fasting Safety: What to Watch For

Fasting, when done correctly, can be safe and beneficial. However, it's vital to be aware of potential risks and warning signs. Here's what to watch for:

- Dehydration: Make sure to stay adequately hydrated, especially during extended fasts. Signs of dehydration include dry mouth, dark urine, and dizziness.

- Electrolyte Imbalance: Prolonged fasting can lead to imbalances in essential electrolytes like sodium and potassium. Muscle cramps, weakness, or irregular heartbeats can be signs of such imbalances.

SLOW DOWN, GO FASTING

- Low Blood Sugar: If you experience severe fatigue, dizziness, or fainting, it could be due to low blood sugar levels. In such cases, it's essential to break your fast and consume a source of glucose.

- Nausea and Vomiting: If you experience persistent nausea or vomiting, it's a sign that your body may not be tolerating the fast well, and you should consider ending it.

- Extreme Hunger and Cravings: While some hunger is expected, if you experience extreme hunger and cravings that are difficult to manage, it may be best to adjust your fasting schedule or method.

In this chapter, we've laid the foundation for your fasting journey, ensuring that you're well-prepared to start your adventure with knowledge, clarity of goals, and an understanding of potential risks. As you continue reading, we'll provide further guidance on how to maintain your fast safely and effectively.

Chapter 8: Fasting in Practice

Daily Fasting Routines - Managing Hunger and Cravings - Incorporating Exercise - Breaking Your Fast: The Right Way

"It is not because things are difficult that we do not dare; it is because we do not dare that they are difficult." — Seneca

You've decided to embark on your fasting journey, and now it's time to put your plan into action. In this chapter, we'll explore the practical aspects of fasting, from daily routines to managing hunger, exercise, and the art of breaking your fast.

Daily Fasting Routines

Daily fasting, also known as time-restricted feeding, is one of the most popular fasting methods. It's relatively simple to incorporate into your daily life. Here are a few key points to consider:

- Choose Your Fasting Window: Determine the hours during which you'll fast and eat. Common windows include the 16/8 method, where you fast for 16 hours and eat during an 8-hour window.

- Stay Hydrated: While fasting, make sure to stay well-hydrated by drinking water, herbal teas, or other non-caloric beverages.

- Track Your Progress: Consider keeping a fasting journal to monitor your fasting periods, meals, and any notable changes in your body and mind.

Managing Hunger and Cravings

Hunger and cravings are natural companions to fasting, especially when you're starting. Here are strategies to manage them:

- Stay Busy: Engaging in activities or tasks can help take your mind off food.

- Drink Water: Often, thirst is mistaken for hunger. A glass of water can curb your appetite.

- Incorporate Filling Foods: During your eating window, choose satiating, nutrient-dense foods to keep hunger at bay.

- Practice Mindfulness: Mindful eating techniques can help you appreciate your meals more fully and reduce cravings.

Incorporating Exercise

Exercise can complement your fasting routine and enhance your results. Here's how to incorporate it effectively:

- Timing Matters: Some people find success exercising during their fasting window, while others prefer to work out during their eating period. Experiment and find what works for you.

- Hydration is Key: During fasts, pay extra attention to staying hydrated, especially if you're active. Dehydration can lead to muscle cramps and decreased performance.

- Listen to Your Body: If you're feeling fatigued or dizzy during exercise, it might be a sign that your body needs nourishment. Consider breaking your fast before your workout in such cases.

Breaking Your Fast: The Right Way

How you break your fast can significantly impact your overall fasting experience. Here are some considerations:

- Start Slowly: Begin with a small, balanced meal that includes protein, healthy fats, and carbohydrates. A good example is a salad with grilled chicken and olive oil dressing.

- Avoid Overeating: It's common to feel ravenous when breaking a fast, but overindulging can lead to discomfort. Pace yourself and eat until you're satisfied, not overly full.

- Stay Mindful: Pay attention to your body's cues. Eating slowly and savoring your food can help you stay connected to your hunger and fullness signals.

- Stay Hydrated: Consider hydrating with water or herbal tea as you break your fast, as your body may be dehydrated after fasting.

In this chapter, we've covered the practical aspects of fasting in your daily life. By understanding how to structure your fasting window, manage hunger, incorporate exercise, and break your fast mindfully, you're better equipped to make fasting an effective and sustainable part of your lifestyle. In the following chapters, we'll continue to explore the many facets of fasting and provide additional guidance to support your fasting journey.

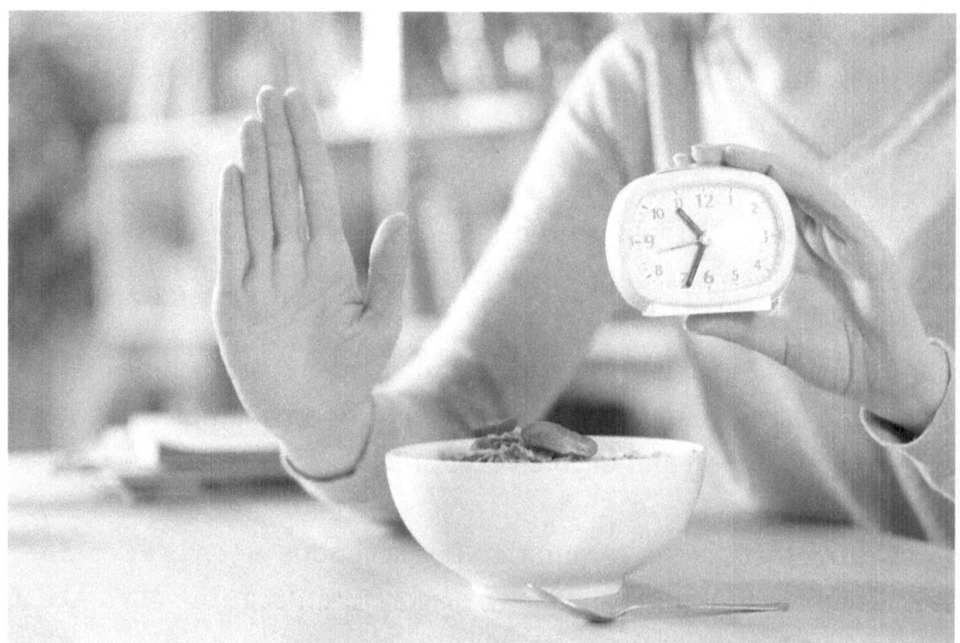

Chapter 9: Common Mistakes and Pitfalls

Overeating During Eating Windows - Neglecting Hydration - Ignoring Nutrient Balance - Fasting for the Wrong Reasons

"The chains of habit are too weak to be felt until they are too strong to be broken." — Samuel Johnson

As you embrace fasting as part of your wellness journey, it's important to be aware of common mistakes and pitfalls that can hinder your progress. In this chapter, we'll explore some of these challenges and how to avoid them.

Overeating During Eating Windows

One of the most common pitfalls of fasting is overindulging during your eating windows. After a period of fasting, it's natural to feel hungry, and this can lead to consuming larger meals than necessary. To avoid overeating:

- Practice Mindful Eating: Slow down and savor your food. Pay attention to your body's hunger and fullness cues.

- Use Smaller Plates: Opt for smaller plates to help control portion sizes.

- Plan Balanced Meals: Plan your meals in advance to ensure they are well-balanced with protein, healthy fats, and carbohydrates.

Neglecting Hydration:

Proper hydration is essential, especially during fasting, as it can help manage hunger and prevent dehydration. Neglecting hydration can lead to fatigue and discomfort. To stay adequately hydrated:

- Drink Water Regularly: Sip water throughout the day, even during fasting periods. Herbal teas and sparkling water can also be hydrating.

- Monitor Urine Color: Clear to pale yellow urine is a good indicator of proper hydration.

- Include Electrolytes: During extended fasts or after intense exercise, consider incorporating electrolyte supplements to maintain balance.

Ignoring Nutrient Balance:

Fasting is not an excuse to neglect your nutritional needs. Some individuals make the mistake of focusing solely on calorie restriction, which can lead to nutrient deficiencies. To maintain nutrient balance:

- Choose Nutrient-Dense Foods: Opt for whole, minimally processed foods that provide essential vitamins and minerals.

- Consider Supplements: If your fasting pattern restricts certain food groups, consult a healthcare professional to determine if supplementation is necessary.

- Monitor Your Health: Regular health check-ups can help identify any nutrient deficiencies that may develop over time.

Fasting for the Wrong Reasons:

Another common mistake is fasting for the wrong reasons. Fasting should be about improving your health and well-being, not driven by unhealthy motivations such as extreme weight loss or self-punishment. To fast for the right reasons:

- Set Health-Focused Goals: Your primary motivation for fasting should be improved health, whether it's enhancing metabolism, mental clarity, or managing specific health conditions.

- Consult a Professional: If you're uncertain about your motivations, consult a healthcare provider or a registered dietitian for guidance.

- Practice Self-Compassion: Approach fasting with self-compassion and a positive mindset. It's a tool for self-improvement, not self-punishment.

Awareness of these common mistakes and pitfalls is crucial for a successful fasting journey. By avoiding overeating, staying hydrated, maintaining nutrient balance, and fasting for the right reasons, you can make the most of your fasting experience and reap its many benefits. In the chapters to come, we'll continue to explore fasting, providing you with additional insights and strategies for success.

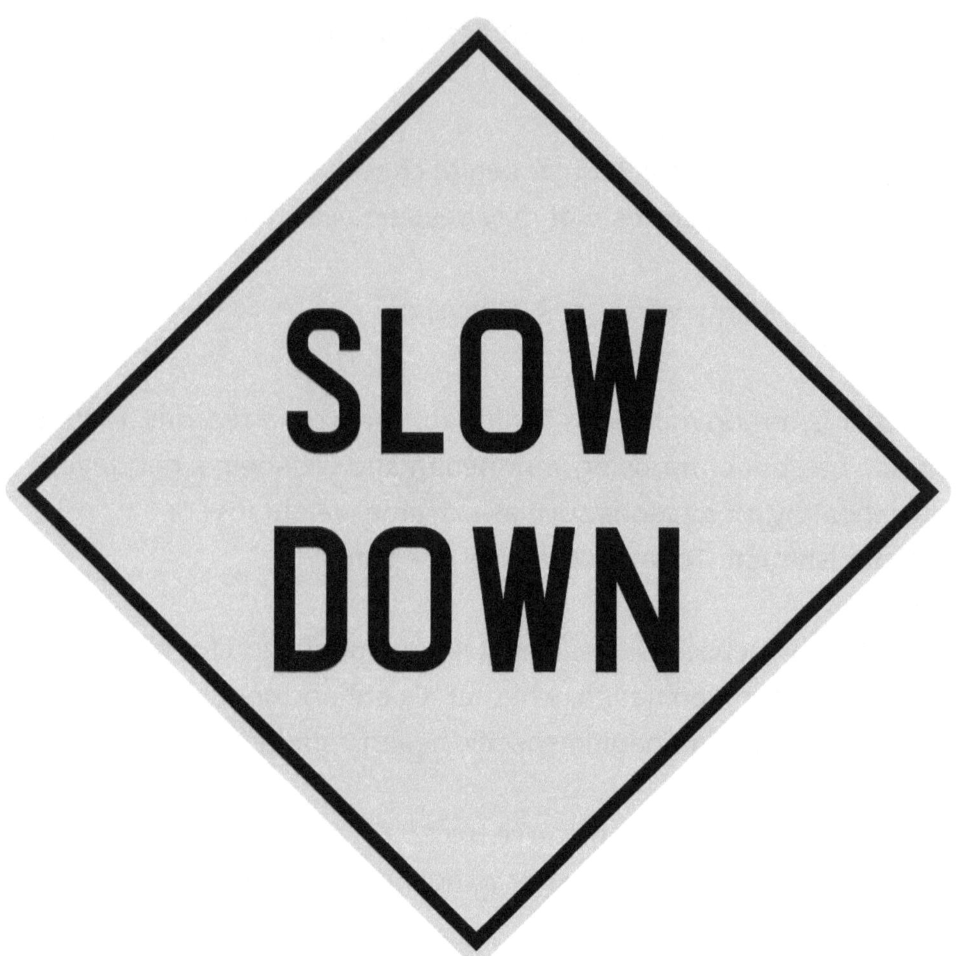
SLOW
DOWN

Chapter 10: Dealing with Fasting Challenges

Social and Emotional Aspects - Plateaus and Stalls - Combining Fasting with Other Lifestyles (e.g., Veganism, Keto)

Many times the rewards of fasting come after the fast, though from time to time answers can come during the fast. -- Jentezen Franklin

Fasting, like any lifestyle change, can present its fair share of challenges. In this chapter, we'll explore some common hurdles you may encounter during your fasting journey and offer strategies to overcome them.

Social and Emotional Aspects:

Fasting can have a significant impact on your social and emotional well-being. Here's how to navigate these challenges:

- Social Gatherings: When dining with friends or family, communicate your fasting schedule in advance. Alternatively, consider socializing during your eating window to share a meal together.

- Emotional Triggers: Stress, boredom, or emotional turmoil can trigger cravings. Practice mindfulness, deep breathing, or engage in a calming activity to redirect your focus.

- Support Systems: Join fasting communities or seek the support of friends or family who understand your goals and can offer encouragement.

Plateaus and Stalls:

Experiencing weight loss plateaus or stalls is common during fasting. Here's how to address them:

- Review Your Approach: Assess your fasting routine and diet. You might need to adjust your fasting schedule or incorporate more variety in your meals.

- Mix Up Your Workouts: If you're exercising, consider changing your workout routine. Your body can adapt to exercise, leading to plateaus. Introducing variety can reignite progress.

- Practice Patience: Weight loss isn't always linear. Your body might be undergoing other positive changes even if the scale isn't moving. Focus on overall health, not just the number on the scale.

Combining Fasting with Other Lifestyles:

Fasting can be combined with other dietary lifestyles, like veganism or keto. Here's how to manage these combinations:

- Vegan Fasting: If you're vegan, focus on plant-based protein sources and nutrient-rich foods during your eating windows. Ensure you get enough protein, iron, and vitamin B12 through vegan sources.

SLOW DOWN, GO FASTING

- Keto and Fasting: Fasting can be compatible with the ketogenic diet, as both involve carb restriction. However, be cautious and ensure your fat intake is appropriate for your energy needs, especially during longer fasts.

- Consult Professionals: If you have specific dietary preferences, consult a registered dietitian or nutritionist to tailor your fasting plan to your lifestyle.

Combining fasting with other lifestyles can be a powerful approach for improving health and well-being. By addressing the social and emotional aspects, overcoming plateaus, and aligning fasting with your dietary choices, you can navigate these challenges and create a sustainable fasting routine that complements your lifestyle. In the chapters ahead, we'll continue to explore fasting and provide you with additional guidance to make the most of your journey.

Chapter 11: The Spiritual Essence of Fasting

The mindful art of fasting, Fasting as a spiritual ritual, My yearly fasting ritual

Fasting is a constant means of renewing yourself spiritually. -- Jentezen Franklin

Fasting is not just a physical practice; it's a profound journey that can have deep spiritual significance. In this chapter, we'll explore the spiritual elements you can incorporate into your fasting routine, from gentle yoga and mindful walking to meditation and music.

The Mindful Art of Fasting:

Fasting, at its core, is a practice of mindfulness. It encourages you to become acutely aware of your body, your thoughts, and your relationship with food. This heightened awareness can be a gateway to spiritual growth. Here are some elements you can weave into your fasting experience:

- Meditation: Integrate meditation into your fasting routine. Use this time to center your thoughts, connect with your inner self, and find peace in the silence of your mind. Meditation can help you uncover a profound sense of spirituality and self-awareness.

- Gentle Yoga: Incorporate gentle yoga sessions to enhance your fasting experience. Yoga can help align your body and mind, promoting a sense of harmony and well-being. The fluid movements and deep stretches can be a beautiful complement to fasting.

- Mindful Walking: Take mindful walks during your fasting period. Whether it's in nature or around your neighborhood, the act of walking with full awareness can be a spiritual practice. Pay attention to each step, the feeling of the ground beneath you, and the sounds of the world around you.

- Music and Mantras: Music can be a powerful tool for spiritual connection. Consider playing calming and spiritual music during your fasting periods. Mantras, repetitive phrases or sounds, can be chanted or listened to, creating a meditative and spiritually enriching atmosphere.

- Journaling: Maintain a fasting journal to document your thoughts, feelings, and experiences. Writing can be a spiritual practice that allows you to explore your inner self and connect with your higher consciousness.

Fasting as a Spiritual Ritual:

For many, fasting is more than a physical practice; it's a sacred ritual. It can be a time of reflection, prayer, or a deeper connection with one's spirituality or faith. Fasting has a long history in various religious traditions and is often used to purify the mind, body, and spirit.

- Intermittent Fasting as a Daily Ritual: Some choose to incorporate daily intermittent fasting as a spiritual ritual. It becomes a consistent practice that helps them stay connected to their faith and spirituality.

- Extended Fasting for Spiritual Purposes: Longer fasts, such as 24-hour or multi-day fasts, can be undertaken with a specific spiritual intention. It's a time for self-reflection, prayer, and a closer connection with one's spiritual beliefs.

- Community Fasting: Fasting in a community, such as during religious observances, can be a powerful spiritual experience. It fosters a sense of togetherness and shared devotion.

Incorporating spiritual elements into your fasting journey can deepen your connection with yourself and the world around you. Fasting becomes more than a physical transformation; it becomes a path to self-discovery and spiritual growth. By embracing mindfulness, yoga, meditation, and music, you can infuse your fasting practice with a profound spiritual essence. In the upcoming chapters, we'll continue to explore fasting, providing you with further insights and guidance for a holistic and enriching journey.

My Christmas Fasting Ritual: Chakra fasting

 My personal yearly Journey of Chakra Transformations through fasting and meditation.

In the midst of the holiday season, when the world is ablaze with the festive spirit, I embark on a unique and deeply spiritual journey. This ritual has become a cherished tradition in my life, where my last meal of the year, shared on the eve of December 25th, marks the beginning of a seven-day fasting pilgrimage.

Each day of this sacred fasting journey is a testament to the power of renewal, guided by the wisdom of the chakras. From root to crown, I dedicate every day to the alignment and cleansing of these energy centers, allowing their vibrant energies to flow freely within me.

Day 1: The Root Chakra (Muladhara) - Red
As I enter this fasting experience, I ground myself in the strength of the root chakra. With the color red as my guide, I establish a foundation of stability and security. I meditate on thoughts of survival, and I explore the art of setting intentions. The journey begins, and I am rooted in my purpose.

Day 2: The Sacral Chakra (Svadhisthana) - Orange
With the energy of the sacral chakra, represented by the color orange, I embrace creativity and sensuality. I cleanse and unlock my passions, dive into the ocean of emotions, and express myself through art. Each brush stroke or stroke of the pen is a dance of emotions.

Day 3: The Solar Plexus Chakra (Manipura) - Yellow
The color yellow radiates from the solar plexus, and I bask in the warmth of self-confidence and personal power. My thoughts focus on empowerment, and I channel this energy into art, creating pieces that reflect the strength within me.

Day 4: The Heart Chakra (Anahata) - Green
With the heart chakra's serene green light, I dive deep into the pool of compassion and love. I journal about gratitude and love for

others and create art that symbolizes the connections that make life beautiful.

Day 5: The Throat Chakra (Vishuddha) - Blue
The clear blue energy of the throat chakra inspires truthful communication and self-expression. I write my innermost thoughts and use colors to convey my emotions. Art becomes a medium for genuine self-expression.

Day 6: The Third Eye Chakra (Ajna) - Indigo
On the sixth day, the indigo light of the third eye chakra illuminates my inner wisdom and intuition. My thoughts center on clarity and insight, and my art becomes a reflection of the visions that guide me.

Day 7: The Crown Chakra (Sahasrara) - Violet or White
As I conclude this fasting journey, the crown chakra, adorned with the colors of violet or white, connects me to the divine. I meditate on oneness and higher consciousness, and my art transcends the earthly plane, conveying spiritual experiences beyond words.

Throughout these seven days, I carry with me an assortment of crystals, each attuned to the chakra of the day. Their energies resonate with my intention, creating a harmonious synergy between the physical and spiritual realms.

This fasting ritual is a testament to the power of self-discovery and inner transformation. It is a spiritual odyssey, marked by colors, crystals, art, and introspection. As the final hour of the year approaches, I stand before a new beginning, cleansed, renewed, and ready to embrace the beauty of the world with the energy of my aligned chakras.

SLOW DOWN, GO FASTING

This Christmas fasting ritual is not just a tradition; it is a profound journey of the soul, guiding me towards greater self-awareness and spiritual enlightenment. As I conclude this fasting experience, I am reborn, ready to face the year ahead with a heart full of love and a soul resonating with the vibrant energy of the chakras.

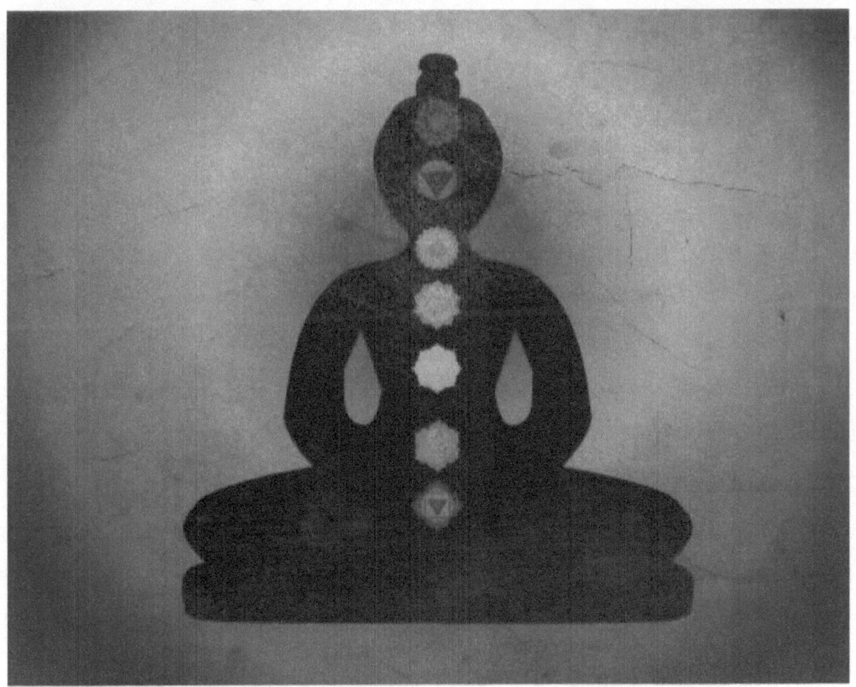

Chapter 12: Fasting for addictions

The everyday addictions, the visible and invisible addictions, unlocking freedom from addictions through fasting,

"Nature cures, not the physician." — Hippocrates

Modern life has introduced a variety of invisible addictions that many of us may indulge in without realizing the extent of their impact. Here are some examples:

1. Smartphone Addiction: Excessive use of smartphones, including social media, gaming, and compulsive checking of notifications, can lead to reduced productivity, disrupted sleep, and increased stress.

2. Social Media Addiction: The constant need to check and engage with social media platforms can result in negative self-comparisons, anxiety, and excessive screen time.

3. Workaholism: An obsession with work and a compulsion to be constantly connected to work-related tasks can lead to burnout, strained relationships, and adverse physical and mental health effects.

4. Online Shopping Addiction: The ease of online shopping and the thrill of purchasing items can lead to financial problems, clutter, and emotional distress.

5. Gaming Addiction: Excessive video gaming, especially online multiplayer games, can result in poor academic or work performance, disrupted sleep patterns, and decreased social interaction.

6. Caffeine Addiction: Overconsumption of caffeinated beverages like coffee, energy drinks, or soda can lead to insomnia, jitters, and dependency on caffeine to stay alert.

7. Sweets and Desserts: A craving for sugary treats can contribute to weight gain, obesity, and an increased risk of chronic health conditions like diabetes.

8. Fast Food Addiction: Frequent consumption of fast food high in salt, sugar, and unhealthy fats can lead to poor nutrition, obesity, and various health issues.

9. Streaming and Binge-Watching: The binge-watching culture, driven by platforms like Netflix, can lead to sedentary behavior, reduced productivity, and disrupted sleep patterns.

10. News and Information Overload: Constantly checking news and information sources, often driven by the fear of missing out (FOMO), can lead to anxiety and information overload.

11. Alcohol or Cannabis Dependency: Frequent and excessive alcohol or cannabis consumption can result in dependency and a range of physical and mental health problems.

12. Prescription Medication Dependency: Over Reliance on prescription medications, especially those with addictive properties, can lead to dependence and potential misuse.

It's important to note that not everyone who engages in these behaviors will develop an addiction. However, if you find that any of these activities are significantly interfering with your daily life, well-being, or ability to manage your responsibilities, it's essential to seek support or professional help to address any potential addiction-related concerns.

Unlocking Freedom from Addiction through Extended Fasting:

Breaking free from addictions, whether they're related to fast food, gaming, or excessive media consumption, is a profound journey. Extended fasting can be a transformative tool on this path to liberation. Here's how it works:

1. Reconnecting with True Needs and Feelings:
  - After a few days of fasting, your body begins to shift its focus. With the absence of regular food intake, it tunes into your true needs, and the artificial cravings tied to addictions start to unravel.
  - The detoxification process that occurs during fasting also extends to the mind. As your body clears away the remnants of unhealthy habits, your mental state becomes more serene and focused.

2. Silence and Reflection:
  - Extended fasting creates a space for silence and contemplation. It's like turning off the noise from the outside world and switching on the inner light. This shift in focus encourages self-reflection and self-awareness.
  - In the stillness of fasting, you become more attuned to your emotions, thoughts, and triggers that drive your addictive

behaviors. This heightened awareness is a crucial step in addressing and overcoming addiction.

3. Resetting the System:
   - Just as your body undergoes a detoxification process during fasting, your mind also undergoes a reset. Fasting disrupts the neural pathways associated with addiction, allowing them to weaken.
   - Over time, the intense cravings for addictive substances or behaviors subside, making it easier to break free from them.

4. Enhanced Self-Control:
   - Extended fasting is a testament to your willpower and self-control. Successfully completing a 5 to 7-day fast demonstrates your capacity to set goals, stick to them, and overcome challenges.
   - This newfound self-discipline can be channeled into resisting addictive behaviors once the fast is over.

5. Shifting Priorities:
   - Fasting provides a window of opportunity to reassess your priorities. As you abstain from the addictive substances or behaviors, you gain a clearer perspective on what truly matters in your life.
   - This shift in focus can help you realign your goals with your values, making it less appealing to indulge in harmful addictions.

6. Rebuilding a Healthier Relationship:
   - Extended fasting offers a unique chance to break the cycle of addiction and rebuild a healthier relationship with your body and mind.

SLOW DOWN, GO FASTING

- As you reintroduce food or media consumption after a successful fast, you can do so mindfully, making choices that are in harmony with your well-being.

In summary, extended fasting serves as a powerful catalyst for breaking free from addictions by allowing you to reconnect with your true needs, fostering self-awareness, and weakening the grip of cravings. It's an opportunity for self-discovery, self-discipline, and personal growth that can pave the way for a healthier, addiction-free lifestyle.

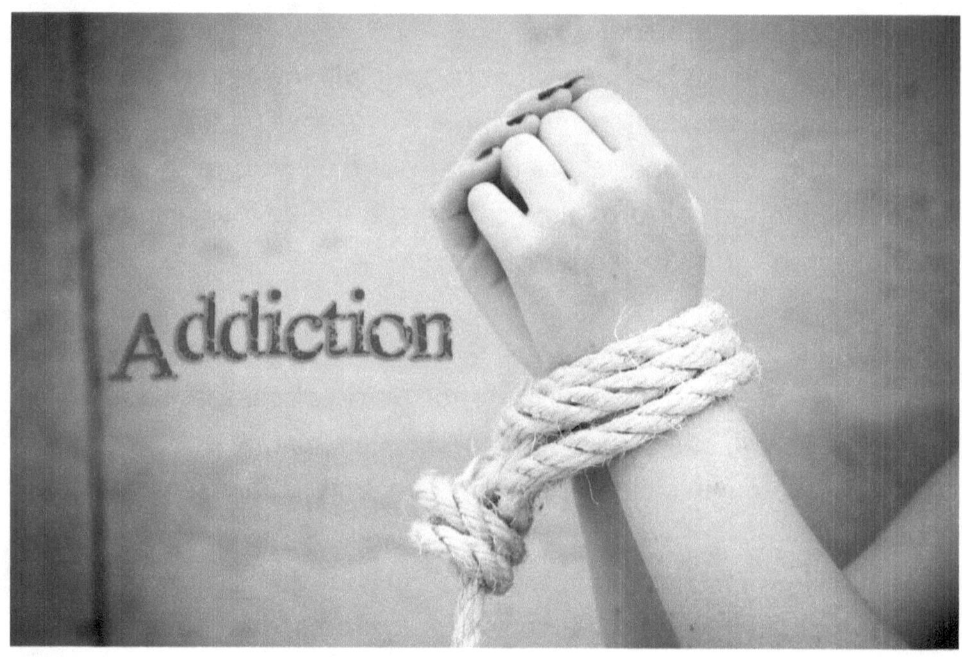

Chapter 13: Personal Stories and Successes

Fasting is a deeply personal journey, and it's always inspiring to hear about the real-life experiences, experiments, and success stories of individuals who have embarked on their fasting journeys. In this chapter, we'll delve into personal accounts, scientific experiments, testimonials, and case studies to showcase the diverse and transformative nature of fasting.

Real-Life Experiments and Scientific Studies:

Fasting has piqued the interest of researchers and scientists worldwide. Real-life scientific experiments have shed light on the physiological and psychological effects of fasting. Here are some noteworthy examples:

- Yoshinori Ohsumi's Nobel Prize-Winning Autophagy Study: In 2016, Yoshinori Ohsumi was awarded the Nobel Prize in Physiology or Medicine for his groundbreaking research on autophagy, a process significantly stimulated during fasting. His work has unveiled the profound cellular benefits of fasting.

- Time-Restricted Feeding Studies: Numerous studies have explored time-restricted feeding (a form of intermittent fasting) and its effects on weight management, metabolic health, and more. These experiments demonstrate the real-world benefits of implementing fasting into daily life.

Testimonials from Fasting Practitioners:

Hearing the stories of individuals who have experienced the transformative power of fasting can be incredibly motivating. Here are some testimonials from fasting practitioners:

- Sarah's Weight Loss Journey: Sarah, a mother of two, struggled with her post-pregnancy weight. After incorporating intermittent fasting into her life, she lost 30 pounds over the course of a year. Sarah found that fasting not only helped her shed the weight but also provided her with newfound confidence and a sense of control over her health.

- John's Mindfulness and Mental Clarity: John, a busy professional, was constantly dealing with stress and a racing mind. Intermittent fasting became a tool for him to find moments of peace and mental clarity during his busy workdays. He credits fasting for his enhanced focus and emotional balance.

- Lisa's Journey to Wellness: Lisa, who had struggled with digestive issues for years, turned to fasting as a way to give her gut a much-needed break. After several juice fasting cycles, Lisa noticed a significant improvement in her digestive health. She emphasizes that fasting was a catalyst for her wellness journey.

Case Studies of Health Improvements

Fasting has also shown its potential as a complementary approach to health management. Here are a few case studies highlighting its impact:

- Case Study: Diabetes Management: A middle-aged man with type 2 diabetes struggled to control his blood sugar levels with medications. After consulting a healthcare provider, he incorporated intermittent fasting into his daily routine. Over time, his blood sugar levels improved, and he was able to reduce his medication dosage.

- Case Study: Weight Loss and Autoimmune Disease: A woman with an autoimmune disease experienced significant weight gain due to her condition. Under medical supervision, she adopted a fasting mimicking diet. Over a period of several months, she lost weight and reported reduced inflammation and joint pain, ultimately improving her quality of life.

These real-life accounts and case studies illustrate the diverse ways in which fasting can positively impact health and well-being. They provide tangible evidence of how fasting can be tailored to individual needs and lead to transformative results. Whether for weight loss, mental clarity, health management, or spiritual growth, fasting offers a world of possibilities. In the final chapters of this book, we'll explore additional aspects of fasting, offering you a comprehensive guide to your fasting journey.

Fasting for Change: The Legacy of Gandhi

Mahatma Gandhi, the great Indian leader and philosopher, is often celebrated for his unwavering commitment to nonviolence, social justice, and his pivotal role in India's struggle for independence

SLOW DOWN, GO FASTING

from British colonial rule. However, it is through his remarkable use of fasting as a tool for change that we witness the true extent of his heroism and his indelible impact on history.

Gandhi's fasting was not a passive act of self-denial but a powerful form of protest and civil disobedience. He believed that by willingly subjecting himself to suffering through fasting, he could awaken the moral conscience of his oppressors and inspire change. His fasts were a testament to the power of the human spirit and the profound impact one individual could have on the course of history.

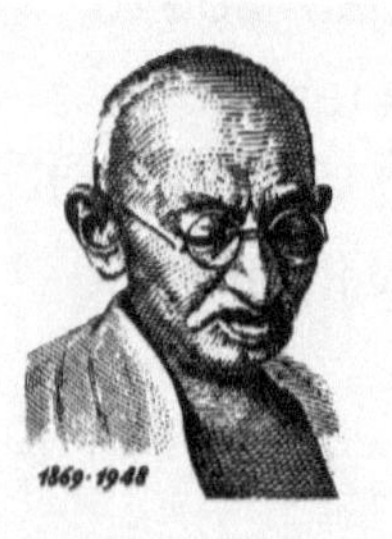

In this chapter, we delve into the extraordinary stories of Gandhi's fasts, each one a symbol of his determination to right the wrongs of the world. From the Salt March to the famous fasts unto death, Gandhi's use of fasting as a political weapon challenged the status quo, shook empires, and inspired millions.

We explore the deep spiritual underpinnings of his fasting practices, the physical and emotional toll they took, and the remarkable outcomes they achieved. Gandhi's legacy serves as a timeless reminder that even in the face of the greatest adversity, one person's unwavering commitment to justice can alter the course of history. His life is a testament to the enduring power of fasting as a catalyst for change and a source of profound inspiration.

One of the most iconic and impactful instances of Gandhi's fasting in India's struggle for independence was the Salt March, also known as the Dandi March, which took place in 1930. This event demonstrated the transformative power of nonviolent resistance and fasting.

The salt march:

At that time, the British government had imposed a salt tax on Indian citizens, making it illegal for them to produce or collect salt, a commodity essential for daily life. This unjust tax disproportionately burdened the poor, who relied on salt as a basic necessity.

In response, Mahatma Gandhi decided to lead a 240-mile march from his Sabarmati Ashram to the coastal town of Dandi, Gujarat. He embarked on this journey with 78 of his followers. The objective was simple yet profound: to make their own salt from the seawater at Dandi, thus defying the British monopoly on salt production and distribution.

Gandhi's message was clear: nonviolent civil disobedience could challenge British authority, and fasting was his means of conveying the urgency of this message. As he marched, he did not eat, but he continued to address the crowds that gathered along the way. Gandhi's determination and the peaceful nature of the protest inspired millions of Indians.

The Salt March captured the world's attention. As Gandhi and his followers reached Dandi on April 6, 1930, they began to make salt by evaporating seawater. This act of defiance demonstrated the power of ordinary people to challenge oppressive laws and the British Empire itself.

The response was swift and significant. Protests and civil disobedience spread throughout India, leading to mass arrests. The global press covered the events extensively, putting international pressure on the British government. Gandhi's symbolic fasting during this time conveyed his commitment to the cause.

SLOW DOWN, GO FASTING

In the face of widespread unrest and mounting international criticism, the British government was forced to negotiate with Indian leaders. In 1931, the Gandhi-Irwin Pact was signed, leading to the release of political prisoners and the representation of Indian leaders at the Second Round Table Conference in London.

Though full independence was not immediately achieved, the Salt March and Gandhi's fasting had set in motion a series of events that ultimately led to India's independence in 1947. Gandhi's unwavering commitment to nonviolence, his powerful symbolism of fasting, and his dedication to justice played an instrumental role in dismantling the British Empire and securing India's freedom. This historic episode remains a testament to the effectiveness of nonviolent resistance and fasting as tools of change.

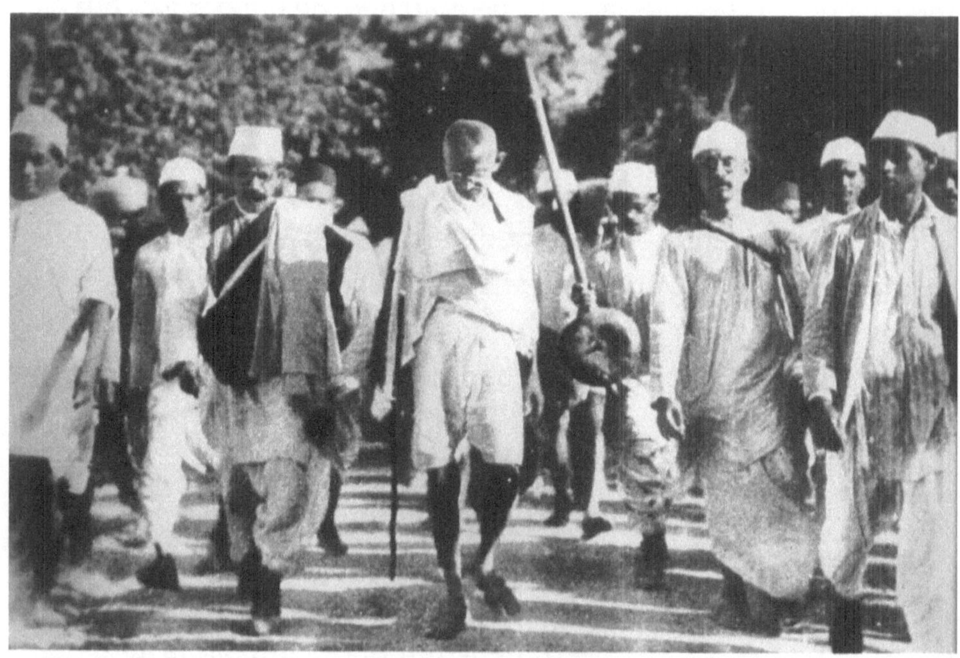

Chapter 14: Breatharianism, Nourishing the Body with Air and Light

"Breatharianism is not about starving the body; it's about nourishing the spirit." — Ellen Greve (Jasmuheen)

The world of fasting encompasses a wide range of practices, some of which challenge conventional norms and beliefs. Among these unconventional fasting methods is the Breatharian lifestyle—a practice that goes beyond traditional fasting by eliminating food and sometimes even water from one's diet entirely. In this chapter, we delve into the fascinating world of Breatharianism, exploring the claims, controversies, and the individuals who choose to embrace a life without eating.

Breatharianism is a lifestyle based on the belief that individuals can sustain themselves solely on air, sunlight, and, in some cases, cosmic energy. Followers of this practice maintain that the human body can draw all the necessary nutrients and sustenance from these non-food sources.

Proponents of Breatharianism assert that by harnessing the power of breath and energy, they can transcend the need for conventional nourishment. However, these claims are met with skepticism and concerns about the potential health risks associated with prolonged periods of non-eating.

This chapter explores the personal stories and experiences of individuals who have chosen the Breatharian lifestyle. They share their motivations, challenges, and insights into the profound changes that this choice has brought to their lives.

The Choice of Non-Eating

The Breatharian lifestyle is a fascinating and unconventional fasting approach that raises many questions and discussions. This chapter invites you to explore the world of Breatharianism with an open mind, providing you with insights into the motivations, experiences, and controversies surrounding those who embrace the path of non-eating.

The Breatharian lifestyle is rooted in the belief that individuals can transcend the need for conventional food and subsist solely on air and light, often considered as forms of nourishment beyond the physical. Followers of this practice maintain that the human body has the inherent capacity to draw vital energy and sustenance from the environment, and that this energy is enough to support life and well-being.

Air as Nourishment

In the Breatharian philosophy, air is regarded as a source of prana, chi, or life force energy. Practitioners believe that through conscious breathing and meditation, they can absorb this energy directly into their bodies. It is seen as a means to nourish not only the physical body but also the mind and spirit. While this perspective on air as sustenance is not widely accepted by mainstream science, it forms the foundation of Breatharian beliefs.

Sunlight as Food

Sunlight, or solar energy, is another integral component of the Breatharian lifestyle. Followers maintain that by exposing themselves to sunlight and harnessing its energy, they can fuel their bodies with the essential nutrients required for life. This concept aligns with the idea that sunlight provides essential vitamins, primarily vitamin D, which plays a crucial role in various bodily functions.

Breatharians often emphasize that their practice goes beyond the physical aspects of sustenance. They believe that living on air and light enhances mental clarity, emotional balance, and spiritual connection. It is not merely a diet but a holistic way of life that aims to free the individual from the constraints of physical nourishment.

The Science and Skepticism

Breatharianism is far from mainstream fasting practices, yet it offers a unique perspective on the human body's capacity to adapt and undergo radical changes. We compare and contrast Breatharianism with traditional fasting methods and their well-documented health benefits.
The Breatharian lifestyle is highly controversial and met with skepticism. Many skeptics argue that prolonged periods of non-eating can lead to severe malnutrition, organ damage, and even death. The scientific community largely rejects the idea of

living solely on air and light, as the human body requires a range of nutrients for survival.

Safety and Health Considerations

For those interested in exploring the Breatharian path, it is crucial to consider the potential health risks associated with extreme fasting practices. Medical professionals strongly caution against such practices, emphasizing the importance of a balanced and nutritionally complete diet for overall health and well-being.

It is essential to address the potential health risks associated with Breatharianism. We provide information on the importance of responsible choices and informed decision-making for those intrigued by this lifestyle.

While Breatharianism challenges conventional notions of nutrition and fasting, this chapter aims to present an objective and balanced view of the practice. It offers a comprehensive exploration of the Breatharian lifestyle, the people who follow it, and the implications it has for our understanding of the human body's capabilities.

A Unique Perspective on Sustenance

Breatharianism offers a unique and unconventional perspective on human sustenance. It challenges societal norms and perceptions of nutrition, proposing that the potential for nourishment exists beyond the physical. While the Breatharian lifestyle remains a highly debated and unverified concept, it serves as a thought-provoking exploration of the human body's extraordinary adaptability and the possibility of nourishment beyond what is conventionally accepted.

The organizations mentioned, Pranicenter and Breatharian World, are associated with the Breatharian lifestyle and offer insights, guidance, and resources for those interested in exploring this unique fasting practice.

Pranicenter

Pranicenter is a prominent organization that promotes the Breatharian lifestyle and provides information, workshops, and resources related to non-eating and living on prana, or life force energy. Pranicenter's website offers various courses, retreats, and events where individuals can learn more about the practice, its principles, and practical techniques.

Resources and Workshops: Pranicenter provides access to workshops and training sessions that cover topics such as breatharianism, energy healing, and holistic health. These resources aim to educate and guide individuals interested in the lifestyle.

Community and Support: Pranicenter offers a platform for like-minded individuals to connect, share experiences, and support one another on their Breatharian journey. This sense of community can be valuable for those exploring unconventional fasting methods.

Here is the link to their website: https://www.pranicenter.com/en/

Breatharian World

Breatharian World is another organization dedicated to the exploration of the Breatharian lifestyle. The website provides information on the principles of living on air and light and offers insights into the potential benefits of this fasting approach.

Educational Content: Breatharian World features articles, videos, and testimonials from individuals who have chosen the Breatharian path. This content is designed to inform and inspire those who are curious about this lifestyle.

Online Courses: The organization offers online courses and programs that cover the foundations of Breatharianism, energy work, and meditation. These courses can serve as a starting point for individuals interested in delving deeper into the practice.

Health and Safety Emphasis: Breatharian World places a strong emphasis on health and safety considerations. It encourages responsible and informed decision-making when exploring the Breatharian lifestyle, highlighting the potential risks and importance of medical supervision.

Both Pranicenter and Breatharian World serve as valuable resources for individuals interested in the Breatharian lifestyle. They offer educational materials, community support, and a platform for individuals to explore and discuss this unique fasting practice. It's important for those considering this path to approach it with caution, conduct thorough research, and prioritize their health and well-being.

Here is the link to their website: https://www.breatharianworld.com/

Chapter 15: Fasting and Your Mind

Fasting for Mental Clarity - Mindful Eating Practices - Fasting and Stress Reduction

"Your body can stand almost anything. It's your mind that you have to convince." — Anonymous

Fasting has a profound impact on the mind, offering benefits beyond physical health. In this chapter, we will explore how fasting can enhance mental clarity, the importance of mindful eating practices, and the role of fasting in reducing stress.

Fasting for Mental Clarity:

One of the most noticeable and sought-after benefits of fasting is the enhancement of mental clarity. As you fast, your body transitions from using glucose as its primary energy source to utilizing ketones, which are produced when your body breaks down fat stores. This metabolic shift can lead to several cognitive benefits:

- Improved Focus: Many fasting practitioners report heightened focus and concentration during fasting periods. This mental clarity is often attributed to the brain's utilization of ketones, which provide a stable source of energy.

- Enhanced Brain Function: Fasting promotes the production of brain-derived neurotrophic factor (BDNF), a protein that supports brain health and the formation of new neurons. This can lead to improved cognitive function and memory.

- Emotional Balance: Fasting can help stabilize mood and emotional well-being. Many people experience reduced irritability and a greater sense of emotional balance during fasting.

Mindful Eating Practices:

Mindful eating complements fasting and can be incorporated during eating windows. It's a practice of being fully present while consuming your meals. Here's how to integrate mindful eating into your fasting routine:

- Savor Your Food: Slow down and savor each bite. Pay attention to the taste, texture, and aroma of your meal.

- Eat Without Distractions: Avoid eating in front of the TV, computer, or while multitasking. Focus solely on your meal.

- Listen to Your Body: Pay attention to your body's hunger and fullness cues. Stop eating when you're satisfied, not overly full.

- Gratitude and Awareness: Take a moment before your meal to express gratitude for the nourishment it provides. Be aware of the source and journey of your food from farm to plate.

- Drink often: Drink a lot of water and herb teas throughout our day, Avoid drinking with or too close to the mealtime. Alcoholic drinks shall be taken in moderation.

Fasting and Stress Reduction:

Stress is a common challenge in today's fast-paced world, and it can take a toll on both physical and mental health. Fasting can be a powerful tool for stress reduction:

- Cortisol Regulation: Fasting can help regulate cortisol levels, the stress hormone. It prevents the excessive release of cortisol, reducing the body's stress response.

- Mental Resilience: Fasting may enhance mental resilience, making you better equipped to handle stressors. This is partly attributed to the brain-boosting effects of ketones.

- Relaxation and Mindfulness: Fasting periods provide an opportunity for relaxation and mindfulness. Use these moments to engage in deep breathing exercises, meditation, or simply reflect on your day.

- Spiritual Connection: Fasting can deepen your spiritual connection, offering solace and tranquility during challenging times.

Incorporating these elements into your fasting routine can significantly enhance your mental well-being. Fasting promotes mental clarity, and mindful eating practices ensure that you're fully present during your meals. Additionally, fasting can play a vital role in reducing stress and fostering emotional balance. As you continue your fasting journey, remember that it offers not only physical but also mental and emotional benefits. In the final chapter, we'll recap

SLOW DOWN, GO FASTING

the key takeaways from this book and provide guidance for maintaining a sustainable and fulfilling fasting practice.

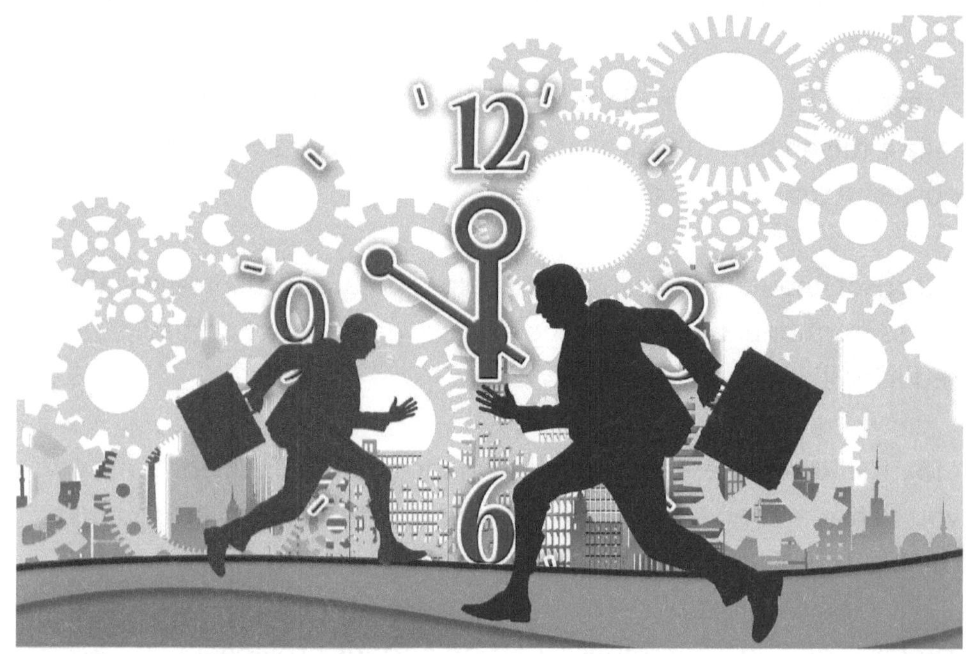

Chapter 16: Fasting for Healing

Fasting for Specific Health Conditions (e.g., Diabetes, Inflammation) - Fasting and the Immune System - Combining Fasting with Traditional Medicine

The best of all medicines is resting and fasting-- Benjamin Franklin

Fasting has been recognized as a powerful tool for healing various health conditions and supporting the immune system. In this chapter, we'll explore how fasting can be used for specific health conditions, its impact on the immune system, and the potential of combining fasting with traditional medicine.

Fasting for Specific Health Conditions:

Fasting can be an adjunct or complementary approach for managing and even improving specific health conditions. Here are a few examples:

- Diabetes: Fasting, particularly intermittent fasting, can enhance insulin sensitivity and help manage blood sugar levels. It's important for individuals with diabetes to consult healthcare professionals when incorporating fasting into their management plan.

- Inflammation: Chronic inflammation is linked to various health issues, including arthritis and cardiovascular diseases. Fasting, especially fasting mimicking diets, has been shown to reduce inflammation markers and can be beneficial for those dealing with inflammatory conditions.

- Autoimmune Diseases: Fasting mimicking diets, which provide essential nutrients at reduced calorie levels, may alleviate symptoms of certain autoimmune diseases. Always consult with a healthcare provider before attempting this approach.

- Obesity: Fasting can be an effective tool for weight management, which, in turn, can alleviate various obesity-related health conditions, including sleep apnea and high blood pressure.

Fasting and the Immune System:

Fasting can have a profound impact on the immune system, potentially enhancing its function. Some key points to consider:

- Cellular Autophagy: Fasting stimulates cellular autophagy, a process that helps remove damaged cells and support immune system health. This cellular "cleanup" may contribute to improved immune function.

- Stem Cell Regeneration: Periodic fasting has been linked to the regeneration of new immune cells, which can strengthen the immune system and improve its ability to defend against infections.

- Reduced Inflammation: By reducing chronic inflammation, fasting may also lessen the burden on the immune system, allowing it to focus on more immediate threats.

- Immune Tolerance: Fasting may promote immune tolerance, reducing the risk of autoimmune reactions.

Combining Fasting with Traditional Medicine:

It's important to emphasize that fasting should be viewed as a complementary approach to traditional medicine rather than a replacement. Here are some considerations for combining fasting with traditional medical care:

- Consult Healthcare Professionals: Always consult with healthcare providers before starting a fasting regimen, especially if you have underlying health conditions or are taking medications.

- Regular Monitoring: When using fasting to manage health conditions, it's essential to monitor your progress and stay in close communication with your healthcare team.

- Medication Adjustments: If fasting leads to significant health improvements, you may need adjustments to your medication or treatment plan. This should only be done under professional supervision.

- Customized Approaches: Traditional medicine and fasting can be customized to work synergistically for individual health needs.

By combining fasting with traditional medicine and medical guidance, you can optimize your approach to healing and overall health. Fasting offers the potential to support healing in various health conditions, boost the immune system, and promote overall well-being. As we conclude this book, we'll recap the key takeaways and provide guidance for maintaining a sustainable and fulfilling fasting practice.

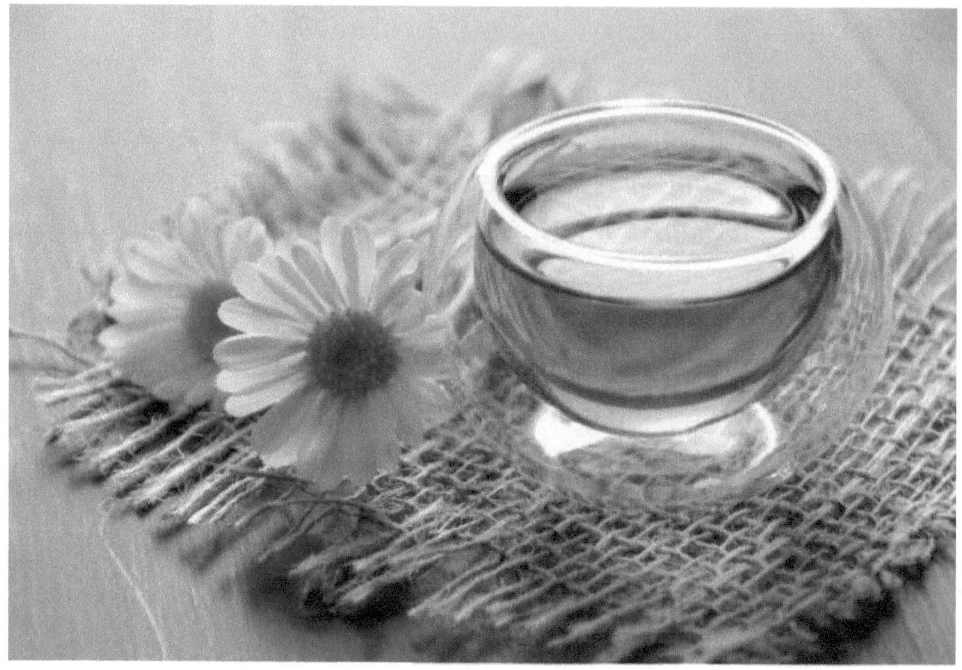

Chapter 17: Incorporating Fasting into Your Lifestyle

Long-Term Fasting Strategies - Fasting and Sustainability - Fasting for Life: Lessons and Takeaways

"Fasting is the greatest remedy—the physician within." — Paracelsus

As you've journeyed through the previous chapters, you've gained insights into the diverse facets of fasting. In this concluding chapter, we'll explore long-term fasting strategies, the sustainability of fasting, and share valuable lessons and takeaways for making fasting an integral part of your lifestyle.

Long-Term Fasting Strategies:

Fasting can be a lifelong practice when approached thoughtfully. Consider these strategies for integrating fasting into your long-term lifestyle:

- Consistency: Maintain a consistent fasting routine that aligns with your goals and lifestyle. Whether it's daily intermittent fasting or periodic extended fasts, consistency is key.

- Flexibility: Be open to adjusting your fasting schedule as your life circumstances change. What works at one point may need modification over time.

- Variety: Experiment with different fasting methods. This can prevent monotony and keep your body adaptable to change.

- Professional Guidance: If fasting for specific health conditions, consider working with healthcare professionals who can provide guidance and monitor your progress.

- Fasting Community: Engage with a fasting community or support network. Sharing experiences and learning from others can be motivating and enlightening.

Fasting and Sustainability:

Sustainability is a critical aspect of any lifestyle change. Fasting is no exception. Here's how to ensure your fasting practice is sustainable:

- Balanced Nutrition: When you eat, focus on nourishing your body with balanced, nutrient-dense meals. This ensures you receive essential vitamins and minerals.

- Listen to Your Body: Pay attention to your body's signals. If you feel fatigued, overly hungry, or unwell, it might be time to reassess your fasting routine.

- Enjoyment and Satisfaction: Make sure your eating periods are enjoyable. Savor your meals, and include foods you love while maintaining a healthy balance.

- Long-Term Goals: Identify your long-term goals for fasting. These might include weight maintenance, enhanced mental clarity, or continued health improvements.

- Moderation: Avoid excessive fasting, as this can lead to negative consequences. Balance is key to long-term sustainability.

Fasting for Life: Lessons and Takeaways

As you embark on your lifelong fasting journey, here are some valuable lessons and takeaways to consider:

- Fasting is Personal: Your fasting journey is unique. What works for someone else may not work for you. Adapt fasting to your individual needs and preferences.

- Health First: Prioritize your health when fasting. Consult healthcare professionals as needed, and make adjustments that support your overall well-being.

- Balance is Vital: Balance is crucial in all aspects of life, including fasting. Balance your fasting periods with nourishing meals and a harmonious lifestyle.

- Mindfulness Matters: Mindfulness can elevate your fasting practice. Be mindful not only of what you eat but also of your overall well-being and the world around you.

- Persistence and Patience: Fasting, like any lifestyle change, requires persistence and patience. Set realistic goals and stay committed to your journey.

SLOW DOWN, GO FASTING

Fasting can be a lifelong practice that enriches your physical and mental well-being. By adopting a sustainable approach and drawing lessons from your journey, you can integrate fasting seamlessly into your lifestyle, reaping its manifold benefits for years to come. As you conclude this book, remember that your fasting journey is a dynamic and ongoing experience, and its rewards are both physical and spiritual.

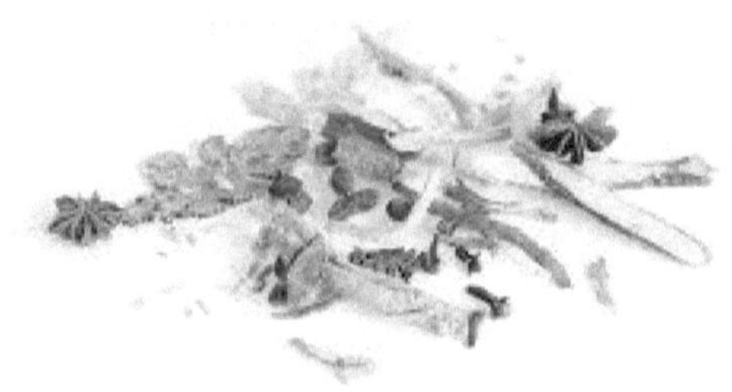

Chapter 18: The Future of Fasting

Ongoing Research and Discoveries - Fasting in Mainstream Medicine - Fasting Beyond the Book: Building a Community

"The future depends on what we do in the present." — Mahatma Gandhi

Fasting, once a niche practice, has gained recognition for its potential to enhance health and well-being. In this final chapter, we'll explore the future of fasting, ongoing research and discoveries, its integration into mainstream medicine, and the idea of building a fasting community beyond the confines of this book.

Ongoing Research and Discoveries

Fasting continues to be a subject of extensive research, yielding exciting discoveries. The future holds great promise for uncovering even more benefits and applications of fasting:

- Fasting and Aging: Research on the relationship between fasting and aging is ongoing. Discoveries in this area may provide insights into extending healthspan and lifespan.

- Fasting and Cancer: Fasting's potential role in cancer treatment and prevention is an active area of study. Fasting mimicking diets and their impact on cancer cells are under investigation.

- Fasting and Mental Health: Fasting's effects on mental health, including its potential to mitigate conditions like depression and anxiety, are being explored.

- Fasting and Regeneration: Research on the regenerative effects of fasting, particularly in relation to organ health and tissue repair, could lead to breakthroughs in medical treatments.

- Personalized Fasting: The concept of personalized fasting, tailored to an individual's unique biology and health needs, may become more prevalent as research advances.

Fasting in Mainstream Medicine:

The integration of fasting into mainstream medicine is gaining momentum. Here's how fasting may become a standard part of medical practice:

- Medical Supervision: Healthcare providers are increasingly incorporating fasting into treatment plans, especially for conditions like obesity, type 2 diabetes, and metabolic syndrome.

- Fasting Clinics: Specialized fasting clinics may become more common, offering medical supervision and guidance to individuals seeking fasting for health and wellness.

- Fasting Prescriptions: In the future, healthcare providers may prescribe fasting regimens as part of comprehensive health management.

- Interdisciplinary Collaboration: Collaboration between fasting practitioners, healthcare providers, and researchers will foster a holistic approach to fasting in healthcare.

Fasting Beyond the Book: Building a Community

Building a fasting community is a vision that extends beyond the confines of this book. Here's how you can contribute to the growth of a supportive fasting community:

- Online Forums and Groups: Engage with online fasting communities, share your experiences, and seek guidance from like-minded individuals.

- Collaborative Events: Consider organizing or participating in events that bring fasting practitioners and experts together. These events can facilitate knowledge exchange and build a sense of belonging.

- Fasting Retreats and Workshops: Explore opportunities to attend fasting retreats and workshops, where you can deepen your fasting practice and connect with others.

- Educational Initiatives: Share your knowledge and experiences with fasting through teaching, writing, or speaking engagements. By educating others, you can foster a more informed and connected fasting community.

The future of fasting is bright, with ongoing research expanding our understanding and the integration of fasting into mainstream medicine providing opportunities for improved health and well-being. By actively participating in fasting communities and engaging in collaborative efforts, you can contribute to the growth and development of the fasting movement. As you look ahead, remember that your journey is part of a broader movement toward a healthier and more balanced future.

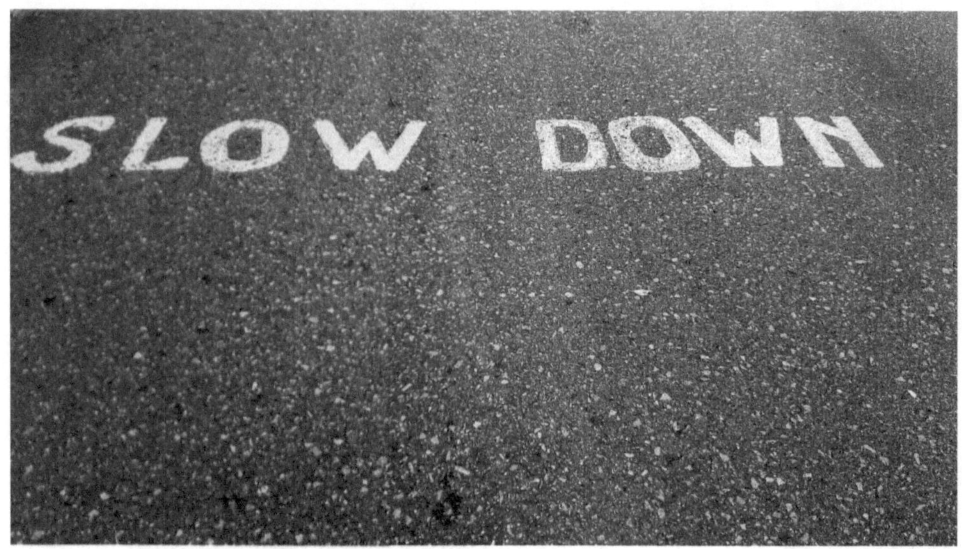

Chapter 19: Conclusion - Reflecting on Your Fasting Journey

Reflecting back on your fasting, Encouragement, the next steps, Final thoughts

"The mind is not a vessel to be filled, but a fire to be kindled." — Plutarch

Encouragement and Next Steps This chapter outline will give you a solid structure for your book on fasting, covering the science, various fasting methods, health benefits, practical tips, and real-life stories.

As you reach the end of this book on fasting, it's time to pause and reflect on your unique fasting journey. In this final chapter, we'll offer encouragement and guidance for your next steps, ensuring that the knowledge you've gained becomes a catalyst for transformative change in your life.

Reflecting on Your Fasting Journey:

Take a moment to look back on the pages you've turned and the knowledge you've absorbed throughout this book. Your fasting journey is a dynamic and personal experience, and it's essential to reflect on your achievements, challenges, and goals. Consider the following:

- Achievements: Celebrate your fasting achievements, whether it's weight loss, improved mental clarity, or better health. Recognize the progress you've made on this journey.

- Challenges: Acknowledge the challenges you've faced during fasting and how you've overcome them. Challenges are opportunities for growth.

- Goals: Revisit your initial goals for fasting. Are they still relevant, or have they evolved? Setting clear goals can provide direction for your continued journey.

- Self-Discovery: Fasting is not just about physical transformation; it's an opportunity for self-discovery. What have you learned about yourself, your body, and your relationship with food?

- Sustainability: Assess the sustainability of your fasting practice. Is it a sustainable and enjoyable part of your lifestyle? If not, what adjustments can you make?

Encouragement and Next Steps:

As you reflect on your fasting journey, remember that it's a path of self-improvement, well-being, and personal growth. Here's some encouragement and guidance for your next steps:

- Stay Committed: If fasting has brought you benefits, whether physical or spiritual, continue to embrace it as a part of your life. Consistency is key.

SLOW DOWN, GO FASTING

- Listen to Your Body: Pay attention to your body's signals and adjust your fasting practice as needed. Flexibility and adaptation are essential.

- Seek Professional Guidance: If you have underlying health conditions, are pregnant, or are taking medications, consult healthcare professionals before continuing your fasting journey.

- Share Your Knowledge: If you're passionate about fasting, consider sharing your experiences and knowledge with others. You can be a source of inspiration and guidance for those beginning their journey.

- Stay Curious: Fasting is a field of ongoing discovery. Stay curious and open to new research and developments in the world of fasting.

As you turn the final page of this book, remember that your fasting journey is a personal and lifelong adventure. The benefits of fasting extend beyond physical health to encompass mental clarity, spiritual connection, and well-being. We hope that the knowledge and insights you've gained from this book continue to enrich your life. May your fasting journey be fulfilling, sustainable, and transformative.

Final thoughts: Embracing the Fasting Journey

As you turn the final page of this book, I hope you are filled with a sense of empowerment and inspiration. Your journey through the world of fasting has been a voyage of discovery, transformation, and renewal. It's not merely an ending; it's the commencement of a lifelong odyssey toward health, well-being, and self-realization.

SLOW DOWN, GO FASTING

Fasting is not just a temporary practice; it's a way of life, an embodiment of the profound connection between your physical body, your mind, and your soul. It's about honoring the wisdom of ancient sages and the courage of those who dared to explore the extraordinary potential of the human spirit.

Through these pages, you've learned that fasting is a path to clarity, both in mind and body. It's a journey that allows you to tap into the hidden reservoirs of strength and resilience within you. It's a means to discover a harmonious relationship with the food you eat, savoring every morsel with gratitude and mindfulness.

As you've explored the science of fasting, delved into the various fasting methods, and understood the profound health benefits, you've realized that your body is an incredible machine, capable of rejuvenation, repair, and transformation. The stories of old sages, monks, and remarkable individuals who fasted as a path to spiritual enlightenment remind us that fasting is more than a physical endeavor; it's a spiritual voyage that connects us to the depths of our souls.

Your journey doesn't end here; it's a continuum. Your fasting practice will evolve and adapt, just as you will. I encourage you to stay committed, be persistent, and remain curious. Listen to your body, for it holds the wisdom you seek. Embrace challenges as opportunities for growth, and celebrate your achievements, no matter how small or grand.

In conclusion, I invite you to reflect on your fasting journey, to rekindle the spark of your initial inspiration, and to set your intentions for the path ahead. As you continue this adventure, remember that your health and well-being are not destinations but ongoing processes. Fasting is a companion on this journey, offering you renewed vitality, mental clarity, and spiritual connection.

May your fasting practice be a lifelong source of empowerment and inspiration. May it lead you to a profound understanding of yourself and the world around you. May it be the path to a life of balance, gratitude, and well-being.

Thank you for allowing me to be a part of your fasting journey. Here's to your health, your growth, and your extraordinary potential.

With warm regards,

Aroonji

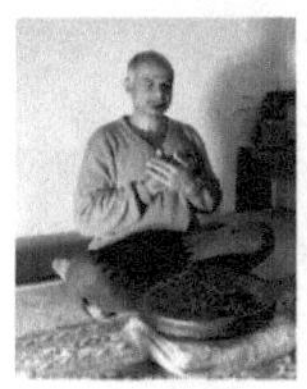

Chapter 20: Interesting Fasting Facts

fasting is a fascinating subject with a rich history and some extraordinary facts and stories associated with it:

1. Longest Recorded Fasting Period: Angus Barbieri holds the record for one of the longest medically supervised fasts. He fasted for **an astounding 382 days,** consuming only water and vitamin supplements. This extreme case highlights the remarkable capacity of the human body to adapt to prolonged fasting.

2. Strange Fasting Phenomena: Fasting can lead to some unusual physical changes. One such phenomenon is known as "ketosis breath." During fasting, the body produces ketones as an alternative fuel source, and their presence can create a distinctive fruity or metallic odor on the breath.

3. Living on Light: The concept of "Breatharianism" suggests that some individuals can live on light and air alone, without the need for traditional sustenance. However, this belief is highly controversial and lacks scientific evidence. It remains a fringe theory, largely discredited by medical professionals.

4. Tales of Old Sages and Monks: Fasting has a deep historical and spiritual significance in many cultures. Monks, sages, and ascetics from various traditions have practiced fasting as a means of purification, spiritual growth, and heightened consciousness.

Fasting played a central role in the lives of historical figures like Mahatma Gandhi and various Christian saints.

5. Fasting and Religion: Fasting is an integral part of religious observances in many faiths. For example, during Ramadan, Muslims fast from dawn to sunset as an act of worship and self-discipline. Similarly, Lent, a Christian tradition, involves fasting and self-denial for 40 days.

These fasting facts and stories highlight the diverse and multifaceted nature of fasting, ranging from remarkable physical feats to profound spiritual practices. While some of these phenomena are extraordinary, they underscore the profound influence of fasting on human physiology, spirituality, and culture throughout history.

Extreme fasting: The Tibetan Monks

 I am personally very intrigued by the discovery of Tibetan monks found in caves, preserved as mummies, which has fascinated researchers and enthusiasts for years. These mummies provide intriguing insights into the practice of fasting and meditation among Tibetan Buddhists, particularly in the context of their pursuit of spiritual enlightenment.

These mummies are often referred to as "self-mummified monks" or "sokushinbutsu." The process of self-mummification was a grueling and extraordinary form of fasting and spiritual discipline. Here's a brief overview of the process:

1. Dietary Restriction: The process began with a strict dietary regimen. The monks would gradually reduce their food intake,

consuming only nuts, seeds, and roots over several years. This was intended to reduce their body fat and prepare the body for mummification.

2. Medicinal Plants: Some monks would also ingest specific types of herbs and plants with antimicrobial properties to help preserve the body during decomposition.

3. Isolation and Meditation: Monks would retreat to remote caves or temple crypts, where they would engage in intense meditation, often in a lotus position. This was believed to facilitate their detachment from worldly desires and to prepare them for the final stages of mummification.

4. Bamboo Tubes: To aid the drying process, monks would drink a special tea made from the sap of the Urushi tree, which acted as a preservative and accelerated dehydration. They would urinate into bamboo tubes to eliminate bodily fluids.

5. Entombment: After their passing, these monks were entombed in a sealed chamber within the cave. Their bodies were often wrapped in cloth or covered in clay to protect them from environmental factors.

The mummies were discovered in a state of remarkable preservation, with skin and hair intact, and are seen as objects of veneration in Tibetan Buddhism. The process of self-mummification represents the ultimate commitment to the spiritual path, as it involves immense physical and mental sacrifice.

These mummies serve as a testament to the incredible lengths to which individuals have gone in their pursuit of spiritual enlightenment through fasting and meditation. They are a living (or rather, preserved) testament to the deep connection between the human body, mind, and spirit in the realm of spiritual practice.

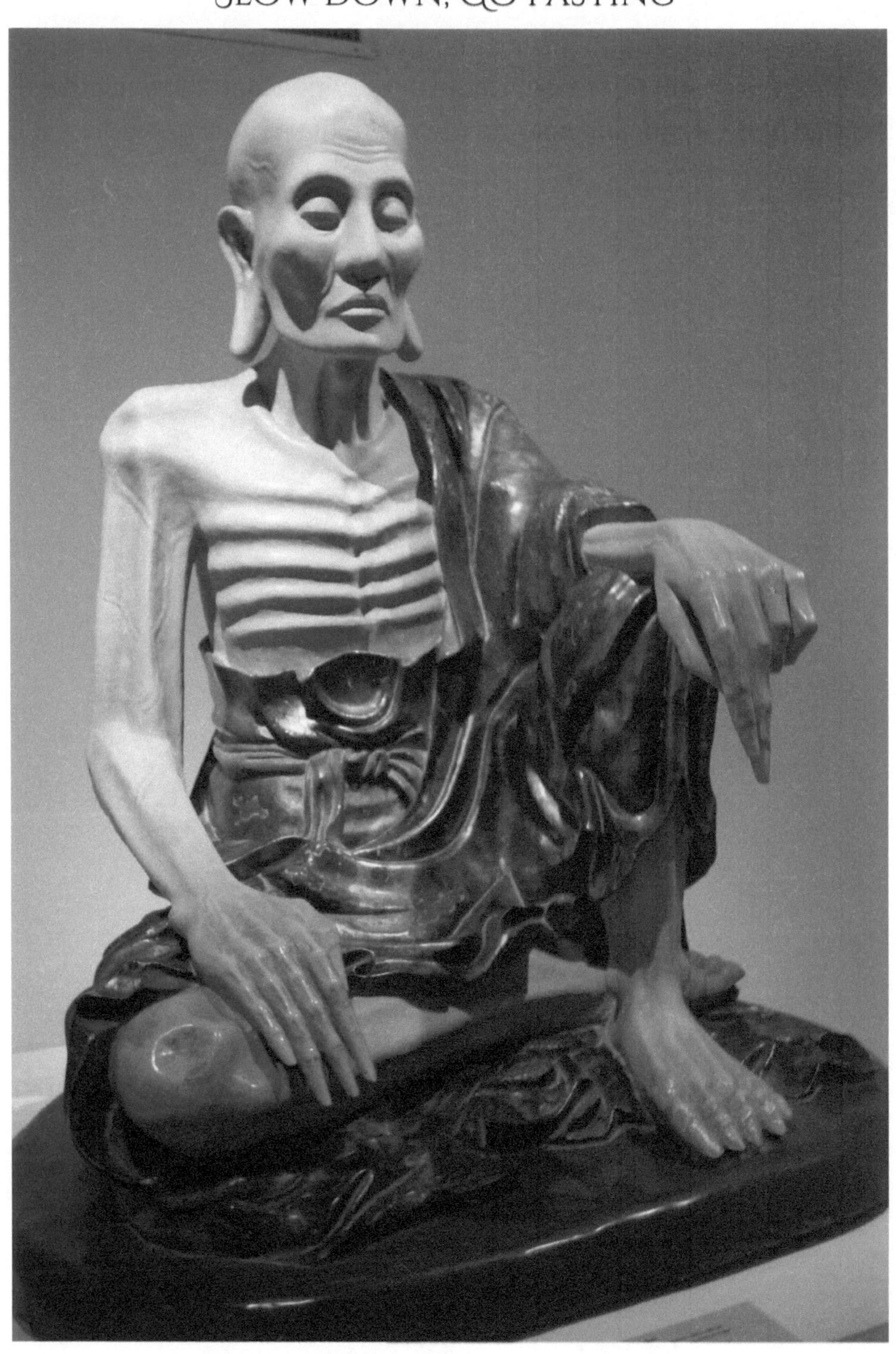

Bonus: Fasting Journal idea!

A fasting journal can be a powerful tool to help readers track their fasting journey, reflect on their experiences, and stay motivated. Here's a creative template idea for an 11-day fasting journal, you need a minimum of three days to see real effects in the body, 11 day is optimum but may be too much for some people, I highly recommend to build it up slowly. you can write your notes here in the book or print out pages. You may start with just one day, then three and slowly build it up.

If you take any medication, or have any health condition, please consult your doctor before starting!

 Each day includes cues and prompts to guide the journaling process:
—------------------------------

Day 1: Starting Your Journey

- Date: _________
- Fasting Method: _________
- Today's Goal: _________
- Thoughts: _________

Reflections:
- What inspired you to start this fasting journey?

- How do you feel as you begin?

Day 2: Embracing the Challenge

- Date: _________
- Fasting Method: _________
- Today's Goal: _________
- Thoughts: _________

Reflections:
- What challenges did you face today?
- How did you overcome them?

Day 3: Discovering Hunger and Satiety

- Date: _________
- Fasting Method: _________
- Today's Goal: _________
- Thoughts: _________

Reflections:
- Describe your hunger and how it changes throughout the day.
- How does it feel to eat when genuinely hungry?

Day 4: Mindful Eating Practice

- Date: _________
- Fasting Method: _________
- Today's Goal: _________
- Thoughts: _________

Reflections:

SLOW DOWN, GO FASTING

- Practice mindful eating during your meal. Describe the experience.
- What did you notice about the taste and texture of your food?

Day 5: A Day of Gratitude

- Date: _________
- Fasting Method: _________
- Today's Goal: _________
- Thoughts: _________

Reflections:
- Begin your meal with a moment of gratitude. What are you grateful for today?
- How did this practice affect your meal?

Day 6: Seeking Mental Clarity

- Date: _________
- Fasting Method: _________
- Today's Goal: _________
- Thoughts: _________

Reflections:
- Did you experience enhanced mental clarity today?
- How did this affect your daily activities and decision-making?

Day 7: Fasting and Energy Levels

- Date: _________
- Fasting Method: _________
- Today's Goal: _________
- Thoughts: _________

Reflections:
- How were your energy levels during the fast today?
- What activities did you engage in, and how did fasting impact your performance?

Day 8: Overcoming Challenges

- Date: _________
- Fasting Method: _________
- Today's Goal: _________
- Thoughts: _________

Reflections:
- Reflect on the challenges you've faced during your fasting journey. How have you grown through these experiences?

Day 9: Fasting and Emotional Balance

- Date: _________
- Fasting Method: _________
- Today's Goal: _________
- Thoughts: _________

Reflections:
- How has fasting influenced your emotional balance and mood?
- Did you find moments of emotional clarity or serenity?

Day 10: Nearing Your Goal

- Date: _________
- Fasting Method: _________

SLOW DOWN, GO FASTING

- Today's Goal: _______
- Thoughts: _______

Reflections:
- As you approach the end of your 11-day journey, what insights have you gained about yourself and your relationship with food?

Day 11: Celebrating Your Achievement

- Date: _______
- Fasting Method: _______
- Today's Goal: _______
- Thoughts: _______

Reflections:
- Celebrate your achievement! What are you most proud of during this fasting journey?
- What are your intentions for incorporating fasting into your ongoing lifestyle?

This creative fasting journal template provides cues and prompts for each day of an 11-day journey. Readers can use it to document their experiences, challenges, and personal insights, making their fasting journey more structured and reflective.
It could easily be adapted for 3 days, 5 days or 7 days fast.

Remember:

"We are what we repeatedly do. Excellence, then, is not an act, but a habit." — Aristotle

Stay Connected, while slowing down

Join Our Fasting Community!

Dear Readers,

I hope you've enjoyed exploring the world of fasting through the pages of this book. Your journey, like mine, is an ongoing adventure, and I invite you to stay connected, share your experiences, and continue our dialogue.

If you have questions, thoughts, or simply want to connect with me personally, please don't hesitate to reach out via email. I'd love to hear about your fasting journey, any insights you've gained, or your thoughts on the book.

fasting@readytoinspire.com or visit my website www.readytoinspire.com for more resources and several online courses for self development.

But that's not all! For an even more vibrant and interactive experience, consider joining our Facebook page dedicated to fasting and holistic well-being. Here, you can connect with like-minded individuals, share your stories, and stay updated on the latest in the world of fasting.

Facebook Group: Slow down, Go Fasting

SLOW DOWN, GO FASTING

https://www.facebook.com/groups/274674362213304/

Joining our Facebook community will provide you with a platform to engage in discussions, access valuable resources, and become a part of a supportive network of fasting enthusiasts.

Your unique fasting journey is an inspiration, and I look forward to connecting with you, sharing experiences, and continuing to explore the profound world of fasting together.

Wishing you health, clarity, and well-being on your fasting path.

A request!

Dear Readers,

I hope you've enjoyed reading my book on fasting and found it both informative and inspiring. Your feedback is incredibly valuable to me, as it helps me understand your thoughts and how this book has impacted your fasting journey.

If you have a moment to spare, **I kindly invite you to leave a review on Amazon.** Whether it's a brief note about what you liked, an insight you gained, or how this book has influenced your approach to fasting, your words can help others discover the benefits of fasting and the joys of this transformative journey.

Thank you for taking the time to share your thoughts. **Your feedback not only encourages me but also guides future readers on their fasting journeys.**

Wishing you continued success and fulfillment on your path to health and well-being.

Warm regards,
Aroonji

"Your body is a temple, but only if you treat it as one."   — *Astrid Alauda*

www.readytoinspire.com